SKIN DISEASE:
A Message from the Soul

CW01096021

SKIN DISEASE:
A Message from the Soul

A Treatise from a Jungian perspective of Psychosomatic Dermatology

Anne Maguire

Free Association Books

Published in the United Kingdom 2004
by Free Association Books
57 Warren Street W1T 5NR

© 2004 Dr. Anne Maguire FRCP (London)

First published in Switzerland in 1991 by
by Walter-Verlag, Olten und Freiburg im Breisgau
titled: *Hauterkrankungen als Botschaften der Seele*
(ISBN 3 530 54408 6)

British Library Cataloguing in Publication Data
A catalogue record for this book is available from the British Library

Produced by Bookchase (UK) Ltd

ISBN 1 853437 48 4
L.D.: SE-3735-2004 in Spain

Printed and bound by Antony Rowe Ltd, Eastbourne

I dedicate this book to Hermes-Mercurius, and to the spirit of Carl Gustav Jung, Franz Riklin and Barbara Hannah.

I also wish to thank most sincerely my brother Michael and my friends Marie-Louise Von Franz and Robert Buissonnière for their unfailing support.

I also give my sincere thanks and gratitude to Nancy and Douglas Thompson who typed the manuscript assiduously.

Of the quicksilver [aqua vitae, perennis] it is said:

"This is the serpent which rejoices in itself, impregnates itself, and brings itself forth in a single day; it slays all things with its venom, and will become fire from the fire [et ab igne ignis fuerit]"

[Tractatulus Avicennae, Art aurif., I. p. 406]
Jung C. G., C. W. Vol 13 para 105 n. 64.

CONTENTS

INTRODUCTION

I THE SOMA

It is perhaps expedient to explore the unique position held by the discipline of dermatology in the medical world.

Medicine is the art and science of healing. It can be further defined as the prevention and alleviation, as well as the cure of disease. Thus it includes the restoration to, and the preservation of, health. As such it is the province of the physician; put quite simply it is doctors' work.

Dermatology is a particular branch of medicine concerned solely with the organ of the skin, and its appendages. Its diseases are treated by those physicians who specialize in the subject, and who are as a consequence said to be dermatologists. In Europe all dermatologists are specialist physicians, who must also understand the entire range of diseases which afflict the human organism. Only dermatologists amongst all physicians regard the skin as a reality in itself and consequently they look at the skin. Non-dermatologists tend usually to look through the skin into the interior of the body where their interests lie. The goal of their search is the disturbed, disordered or diseased internal organ.

Since the interior of the physical body is the true realm of the non-dermatological physician, he tends generally to hold the skin in low esteem, but unfortunately subject to certain incurable, and untreatable diseases.

The individual doctor is not entirely to blame for this restriction of viewpoint. It has been engendered by many factors. Not least of which is the rational intellectualism of the universities which has led to a distinct preponderance of inductive thinking in the medical schools, where only those diseases which appear to have a cause are taken seriously. Since most dermatological conditions appear to be of unknown aetiology, they are easily rejected by the rational intellect as lost causes. There is also the problem of increasing specialization, an ubiquitous malady of the twentieth century. This problem has ramified the discipline of medicine in particular, and led to fragmentation of the science. Even in dermatology itself, the fragmentation process continues, to expand. Another factor which must be considered is the nature of the organ of the skin itself, and which is directly responsible for the collective medical attitude towards it.

This organ is highly complex and quite unique. It is certainly the heaviest in the body. It envelops the entire body and is the chief means of identification between human beings, and is undoubtedly the major organ of sexual attraction. There is also the question of its visibility, it can be observed immediately and in its entirety. Its colour is at once apparent, and its texture is not only seen, but can be felt by the hand to discern and to distinguish the graduations of its singular nature, ranging from the petal softness of a newborn infant's skin, to the resistant granite-like consistency of those who suffer from certain dermatoses the most disfiguring of which are those due to collagen disorders, and the sometimes horrifying genodermatosis of the Darier-White disease.

The skin is the boundary between the internal physical body and the outer world. It is the natural physical limitation of ego consciousness of the individual. Everything beyond the skin is 'other'. Like all boundaries it features both protective and defensive mechanisms.

In health it is a highly stable, and a completely silent organ, emitting not the vestige of a creak or a squeak. In repose it possesses an air of tranquillity and this deceptive quality entices the thought that the skin is eternally changeless. Since in health the skin is calm, quiet, uncomplaining since symptom-free, it requires no attention except a daily devotion to hygiene. It is therefore, generally forgotten or ignored by the vast majority of human beings. In such circumstances it resembles nothing so much as a well-mannered, beautifully domesticated cat, which provided it is kept warm and adequately fed leads a totally independent existence, happily trouble-free for its owner.

But if a dermatosis should arise it is as if the purring cat, becomes a demon of spitting fury. The skin at once loses its tranquillity and often erupts into a blanket of fire, with the appearance of a raging inferno. This is most certainly so with certain disorders such as for example, the urticarias, acute eczemas and dermatitis herpetiformis which can all be hellish tormentors. The image of the skin in totalis, begins to come into focus. It becomes clear as to why it is an organ so easily forgotten, disregarded, or even denigrated. On the other hand it is equally clear that when disturbed it makes its presence felt in no uncertain manner.

The health of the individual human being imparts an extra quality to the skin, which is the summation of a state of tonus, an innate elasticity, and a natural fluctuation of colour. This latter is of course dependent on the constitution of the blood, and the cardiovascular flow at a given time. This specific quality is in its turn also dependent upon the age of the individual concerned.

In particular those numerous appendages of the skin, scalp and body hair, facial hair, and finger and toe nails in similar manner also reflect the underlying state of health of the individual being.

Dermatologists, since they are all physicians, must be concerned chiefly with the physical attributes of disease. An assessment of the physical condition is essential. Occasionally patients present with an apparent skin disease, such as a colour change, although the skin itself is normal, and there is no evidence of disease. The colour change which appears to belong to the skin may ensue from any number of causes, either external to the skin or from an internal disease process. For instance, a yellowing of the skin may appear, which may be due to a simple bronzing effect caused by the sun, or on the other hand it may be due to an obstruction of the biliary circulation, resulting in jaundice. In both instances the skin itself is blameless.

The advent of that commonest of all skin symptoms, pruritus, or itching naturally suggests that the cause is located in the organ itself. Yet maybe it is the result of external parasites, allergy to dust or clothing, or internally the presence of excess bile salts in the blood. It is therefore important for the dermatologist to establish the presence or otherwise of systemic disease in order to ascertain whether or not a skin disorder is primary or secondary, to either an external or internal somatic disturbance.

However the discipline of dermatology is chiefly concerned with those diseases specific for the organ concerned which are not naturally accompanied by underlying physical diseases. Such processes are termed dermatoses. These are legion, and include a large variety of eczemas, all the urticarias, psoriasis, a puzzling and ubiquitous disease, the mysterious lichen planus, and the immensely chronic and sometimes frightening dermatitis herpetiformis, the strangely suddenly erupting disease of pemphigus, and the therapeutically resistant disorders of collagen dysfunction, diseases of the connective tissue, such as lupus erythematosus and scleroderma.

All these, to name but a few, are classed as being of unknown aetiology, and they have proved and still do prove to be an enormous challenge to research in the dermatological field, everywhere. Patients with these disorders are investigated and examined from every physical aspect. The biochemistry of such individuals so affected, is subjected to the closest scrutiny and all modern techniques are utilized to examine and study the composition and the structure of all accessible bodily organs, either in situ via the camera, or the X-ray eye, or by means of surgical investigative procedures. It is true to say that in research centres no cell is allowed to remain undisturbed from the enquiring rational medical intellect. This close scrutiny is certainly intended for the benefit of the individual patient concerned, but

11

there is behind it the attempt also to discover the prime cause of the majority of the aforementioned diseases. To summarize, Ebling[1] "That to understand fully the cause, nature, and treatment of skin disease, requires a knowledge of physiology, structure and chemistry of normal as well as of pathological skin". He also comments "that whilst it may no longer be true to say that skin is a neglected organ it must be admitted that a scientific basis for causation and treatment can be offered to relatively few skin diseases".

During the past forty years medicine has indeed made great progress in all fields, but particularly so in the field of therapy. In dermatology, since the advent of the therapeutic agents the corticosteroids, with facilities for easy and efficacious application topically, the common and widespread eczemas of the past have been aided and controlled for the first time.

Prior to the onset of the regular use of these miraculous drugs, there was untold misery and prolonged chronic suffering, sometimes, lifelong, by those patients with chronic dermatoses, such as the condition of Atopic eczema. It was not at all uncommon for such child patients to remain in hospitals reserved for the chronic sick for periods extending over several years. Furthermore mortality was high due to invasion of the skin by pathological bacterial organisms self-induced by scratching, through the torn and lacerated skin. It was the combination of cortisone and antibiotic therapy which changed the face of dermatology, almost overnight.

Suddenly a new era dawned, and dermatology entered the field of expanding medicine. Research physicians biochemists, microbiologists, and medical scientists of all the varied disciplines began slowly at first and then with increasing momentum to devote their intelligencies and their energies to the problem of the causative factor in the common dermatoses. These disorders presented an unique challenge, because of the visibility and easy accessibility of the skin, and because, and not least, aetiology of most dermatoses was still unknown. The work itself through the years has been painstaking, requiring extraordinary care and has often been brilliant in its exactitude, over the years. It has involved, and indeed continues to do so, all the cell processes of growth and repair, together with the singular activities of respiration, transpiration, and the circulation of the various somatic fluids. Of recent years, a new branch of medicine has appeared, and has rapidly established itself as a foremost newcomer. This is the branch of medical science which has been born anew with the development of transplant surgery. It is concerned with the problem of the immunity of the organism against disease, and the problem of rejection of foreign material by the organism.

Immunology is the term given to the study of immunity, and the immune defence systems. These include those processes by which the body defends itself in order to maintain a constant equilibrium of its internal milieu against invasion by alien organisms or the development of unwanted cells within itself. By such means is the human or animal body protected from the surrounding potentially polluted and therefore hazardous environment.

The subject of immunity naturally includes the search for vaccines but has widened to include the understanding of hypersensitivity states, auto-immune disease, immunodeficiency states, connective tissue disease, and the cancerous state. In all of these the body becomes either hostile towards itself, unable to defend itself, or destructive, towards its own being. Undoubtedly the transplantation surgical technique has not only engendered these new interests, but owes its progress to the establishment of the science of advanced immunology.

From this vast field of research, prodigious information has been supplied towards the understanding of many disease processes producing dermatological manifestations. But alas, in spite of all the effort, the basic cause of the majority of dermatoses has eluded consciousness. In spite of the intensified, as well as the wider increase of interest in this field, no cause has as yet been revealed.

Why is this so? Perhaps there is a certain naïevete in the question. Nature does not lightly yield her secrets. The simple answer to the question is of course, that the unconscious has not yet allowed its secret, viz the knowledge of the causation to be released to scientific medical awareness. The time has not yet arrived for its entry into the rational world. However, perhaps success eludes the researchers, not simply because the question is premature but because the cause of these dermatoses is sought specifically in the somatic realm, where the search is confined to the structure of and the metabolism of the body cell in the physical body.

Perhaps the cause does not lie in that area, perhaps it is elsewhere. Physicians in this modern rational technological age do their doctors' work and such work naturally mirrors the state of society at a particular time period. The physician is therefore closely bound to that very society whose physical health is dependent upon his medical skills. No matter what his status, be it family practitioner, or the holder of a professorial chair, the doctor himself is affected by that very society in which he lives and works.

In the past, the spiritual health of the society was cared for by the religions but since the seventeenth century a great change has overtaken the civilization of Western Christendom. The scientists, replaced the alchemists at that time, and rational intellectualism began to overwhelm the spiritual life of society. The inductive thought and rational explanations of the scientist, informed us that there is no God, and so willy-nilly, the religions have fallen into disfavour and disuse. Sadly the priests themselves have been caught by this pernicious disease of scientific rationalism, and feel that they must themselves likewise explain the great mysteries of life in terms of modern rationalism. Thus they reduce or annihilate the great mystery of the spirit.

It has come to pass that the whole emotional and affective side of man's nature has been thus denigrated, and pushed to the boundaries of conscious existence. In psychic terms it has arrived at an equivalent locus occupied

13

by the skin in its relation to the physical body.

To whom can one turn for an explanation of these strange physical ills which abound today? Ailments whose cause does not lie in the body, or so it seems. In earlier times these ills would have been recognized immediately as belonging to the soul of someone who had erred. Perhaps a mistake had been made, a wrong turn taken, or an evil act performed such as lying, stealing, criminal aggression, the commission of adultery, sodomy, rape, incest, or even murder most foul. All of which acts are not just against society, but more importantly against the innate moral conscience of the individual human being; an act against the soul of the subject. Such a person may be said to have lost his soul, and from which state the illness has arisen. However modern man, and thus society, no longer has the belief in the existence of the soul.

Today, in society at large, there is a great and universal sickness of psyche. Although the initial beginnings are partially obscured, the first great and frightening shudder became apparent in Europe in the French Revolution. It was during this time the goddess of Reason was deified in the cathedral of Nôtre Dame in Paris. The rational intellect severed its connections with the instinctual unconscious, and its ascent began then.

This psychic illness has continued to proliferate with devastating momentum, like a vast fulminating malignancy. It now presents itself, two centuries later in the shadows caused by nuclear dust, with every type of savagery, combined with a world crisis of loss of moral conscience, to the astounded and incredulous gaze of the world.

The physician finds himself face to face with the monstrous barbarism of unconscious forces. Concomitantly he also finds that he is heir to the task, formerly held and recently vacated by the priests. He must concern himself whether he likes it or not, whether he is capable or not, whether he believes it to be true or not, with this immense spiritual problem, since it is thrust upon him. He it is who must confront mental illness, physical disease, and psychosomatic disorders which have erupted in recent years, in spite of all the rational health care, physical ministrations including every type of research provided by various governments and their agencies.

II THE PSYCHE

In the normal course of events, physicians are not taught to consider the soul of man to be their province in the medical schools of their universities. Apart from the psychologists, psychiatrists, medically trained analysts, and psychotherapists few members of the medical profession regard the psyche of man other than with considerable circumspection, that is if they concede its existence at all.

In certain fields considerable speculation rotates around such psychic syndromes as anxiety, depression, stress and tension states in an attempt to relate them to physical disorders. Such plausible rational explanations are in the main, easily acceptable, but by their very nature they further denigrate the psyche of man to a position of secondary importance to the physical body. Even today, the psyche is still considered by many to be an epiphenomenon of the brain.

The word psyche has been in use in the English language since 1647, it is an adoptive of the Greek word psyche for breath, or to breathe, hence it means life, soul, and spirit. The modern meaning is also soul or spirit, as distinct from the body, and since 1658 it has also come to mean the mind.

In later Greek mythology Psyche was personified as the beloved of Eros, the god of love, and was represented as having butterfly wings, or she was sometimes a butterfly. Thus the word means both soul and butterfly. A butterfly is thus symbolic of the soul. 'Psyche' however has a wider meaning than 'soul', in the Christian sense. Speaking generally psyche refers to everything inside, in the inner world, in contradistinction to the outside world.

'Psyche' was for Jung[2] an inclusive term for the totality of all so called psychic processes. He said that all immediate experience is psychic. There is physically transmitted (outer world) experience and inner (spiritual) experience. The one is as valid as the other. He did however state that since[3] "we know from experience that the psyche, can be grasped only to a very limited degree, it would be best to regard it as a tiny conscious world influenced by all sorts of unknown factors lurking in the great darkness that surrounds us."

This leads naturally to the concept of the unconscious. Ego as centre of the conscious mind is a relayer or transmission-communicator. In direct counterstance to ego is the unconscious psyche. In a child the ego complex, which is present from birth gradually and slowly develops out of the unconscious world, like tiny islands arising out of the sea. As the child develops these islets of consciousness aggregate together, and ego is formed, and consolidated much in the same way as the land masses arose out of the primordial ocean, aeons ago.

In the same way man has forged an awareness of himself, as an individual member of humankind distinct from all other species which inhabit the planet. Consciousness is mankind's most precious attribute. It is the light which born from the unconscious, is able to direct itself outwards to the world and inwards towards the realm of the unconscious. Only by being conscious can one comprehend all that which is not, all that which is therefore unconscious. The unconscious is unconscious.

For a moment it may be helpful to examine the development of the concept of unconscious psyche. Great events do not suddenly appear, but slowly evolve over centuries as lesser and greater events occur, to culminate in a transformation of immense importance. For instance at the time of Socrates there existed the atomist theory in which it was thought that the atom was indivisible. In 1945, early one morning in the New Mexican desert, the nuclear theory of the atom was proved incontestably, and exploded forever the former theory in a test explosion of the atom bomb. Although the climax was stupefying in its explosive power an untold number of minds over many centuries had occupied themselves, and worked to achieve the proof that the atom was not indivisible. A transformation had occurred psychically as well as materially, and the world would never again be the same. In one brilliant flash with its following mushroom cloud shadow, the world view was changed for all time.

Immense as was this event, an even greater and vastly more important one has slowly unfolded over the past one hundred and fifty years or so. As with all such psychic transformations the unfolding process is slow and confined to specialist and select circles, thus there is usually no dramatic effect over long periods of time. Receptivity of consciousness to appreciate and integrate the meaning of such developments, is essential. The event to which I refer is the concept of unconscious psyche.

Since the French Revolution, 200 years ago, unleashed the first great unconscious storm, it has never abated. This psychic storm flares up to die down, as war has succeeded war in Europe. The year that the French Revolution started in 1789 a young child was born in Dresden, he was Carl Gustav Carus (1789–1869). He became a professor of gynaecology in 1814, and was known for his learned text books on the subject. Carus was very successful in his medical career, and found his spiritus rector in Johann Wolfgang Von Goethe (1749–1832), German's greatest poet, scientist, and statesman.

From this friendship there developed a certain attitude to nature and to life and he wrote, amongst others, a book called Psyche, published in 1846, in which he describes as he sees it the development of the soul. Carus attempts to hold together the two sides of his own nature, the rational observant practical doctor, and the philosophical idealist.

Before Carl Gustav Carus died Sigmund Freud (1856–1939) was born in Freiberg, in Moravia. He passed eighty years of his life in Vienna. He also qualified as a doctor but specialized in neurology. As a young scientist engaged in biological research, he could hardly have avoided being influenced by the new physics. Energy and dynamics were pervading every laboratory and seizing the scientific mind. Gradually there began to take shape in Freud's mind, the thought that most of these dynamic forces are unconscious. From being a neurologist, he became a scientific psychological investigator. It was the dream which proved to be the door to the unconscious. His work with dreams was to establish the reality of the unconscious.

When Freud was nineteen years old, Carl Gustav Jung (1875–1961) was born in the small village of Kesswil am Bodensee in the North eastern part of Switzerland. Eventually he was to become a doctor of medicine, specializing in psychiatry. He was led to this decision by a chance reading of

Krafft-Ebling's textbook of psychiatry. Intuitively he knew on encountering this book that psychiatry was to become his destined field.

For some years he was closely identified with Freud's school of psychoanalysis. After his break with Freud, he developed his own system, which he called analytical psychology. Apart from treating patients with psychological problems, the system also included a body of concepts and theoretical formulations.

Jung was to ask himself what happened to experiences that failed to gain recognition by the ego? This in fact appears to be a simple question, but in reality is a question of great profundity. For the experiences do not disappear from the psyche, for nothing that has ever been experienced ceases to exist. Instead these experiences which seem to have evaporated into thin air, are stored, in what Jung terms, the personal unconscious. This level of mind is contiguous with the ego. It is the receptacle that contains all those psychic activities and contents which are incongruous to the conscious individuation or function. Perhaps they are conscious experiences which have been repressed or disregarded for all kinds of reasons such as a personal conflict, a moral problem, a disturbing thought, or an unacceptable, (and unconscious) emotion. Often they are simply forgotten because they are unimportant or irrelevant in a life at a certain time. All those experiences which are too feeble to reach or remain in consciousness are stored in the personal unconscious. One important feature of this realm is that its structure is composed of complexes which are groups of contents, aggregated in the form of a constellation around a central nucleus.

It was due to Jung's extensive studies with the word association experiment which first intimated to him their presence.

WORD ASSOCIATION TEST

This test in which the organ of the skin played the vital rôle as psychic mediator was developed by Jung when he worked as a psychiatrist at the Burghölzli Psychiatric Hospital in Zürich at the turn of the century. It was to mark the beginning of his understanding of the psychic material which presented itself to him, in the course of his work, and during his subsequent psychiatric investigations and studies. Between the years of 1904 and 1907 Jung's early work produced the extraordinary and exciting demonstration that the skin's electrical activity changed remarkably when certain specific words, (charged with emotional overtones for the subject) were spoken in the course of the test. It became clear that mental activity particularly the process of recall evoked by simple verbal stimuli was consistently and continuously reflected by skin changes. Jung's[4] paper on his psychological investigations with the galvanometer was originally published in English in a neurological scientific journal.[5] The purpose of this research was to ascertain the value of the so called "psycho-physical galvanic reflex" as a recorder of psychical changes in connection with sensory and psychical stimuli.

Coming events often cast their shadow before, it is interesting therefore to recall the events which preceded the development of the test. In the last decade of the nineteenth century Tarcharoff[6] discovered that the galvanometric phenomena in human skin occurred both with sensory irritation and with various forms of psychic activity. He noted that strong emotions and mental computations, accompanied by emotion, produced deviations in the galvanometer. Throughout the subsequent years, various experimenters, including Galton,[7] and Wündt[8] took up the researches. The latter produced a test called the "association experiment". This consisted of an experimenter calling out a random word to the subject in reply to which, the subject as quickly as possible had to reply with the first word which presented itself to him. A series of pairs resulted, called associations. The called word was known as the stimulus word, and the reply, the reaction. The Wündt school produced others who undertook further investigations. These included Kraepelin,[9] Aschaffenburg[10] and Sommer[11] who missed the essential point of psychic influence in the test, Muller[12] who confirmed Tarcharoff's original work, and Veraguth.[13] The latter was a Swiss neurologist who gave the name of "psycho-physical galvanic reflex" to the phenomenon, and also corroborated Tarcharoff's findings.

Jung it was who suggested to Veraguth that a list of unrelated words was incorporated and pronounced. Then those words connected with some emotional complex, produced an effect on the galvanometer, whilst indifferent words did not have any such reaction. He concluded that only stimuli associated with emotionality induced a deviation in the galvanometer, but he was unable to explain the phenomenon. It was Veraguth who first made known to Jung the value of the galvanometer, as a measure of psychical stimuli. After this demonstration Jung[14] tells us that he began to experiment on his own account the work which Wündt had originated.

As Hannah[15] states, the test had been used before only on lines of conscious thought, and the reason that it is now so often associated with Jung is that he was the first to enquire into the disturbances in reaction thus making it a valuable method of investigating the deeper roots of mental illness. It was this test which was to lead him to a recognition of the existence of the complexes, and to the discovery of the unconscious, independently of Freud. Interestingly enough this remarkable series of described events which led Jung to his subsequent discoveries and momentous conclusions were overshadowed by another and unexpected development.

For every action there is always a counteraction and although as we have observed Jung took the inner exploratory way to unravel the mysteries of human psychic life, at about the same time in Russia, Pavlov opened up another pathway. His principles of conditioning theories of learning swept the experimental psychologists into, the easier, safer, and infinitely less taxing experimentation of human behaviour in animals. A very great change occurred, and a torrent of scientific energy was thus directed towards animal research, and away from human mind research as had been the case before.

Some eight decades later, the scientific study of behaviour has been forcibly directed, almost without exception, towards the physical side of the biological organism. Scientists naturally have been concerned solely with measuring devices in their experimentation of both internal and external events. The inner life of the human subject, his moods, thoughts, feelings, and intuitions could not be titrated, weighed or measured, consequently they were regarded as irrelevant to the experiment. It came to pass that the psyche of man was cast aside, and the physical body assumed the mantle of sovereignty in scientific eyes. Emphasis therefore has veered towards perfection of the ability to control emotion, and behaviour pattern externally. Since the subject is not usually considered as an individual, merely a member of the human race his emotional life must of necessary be at the mercy of these factors. Nowhere is this more evident than in the scientific discipline of medicine, in which, the psyche of man should have been given its rightful, central place. Alas, the compassi medicii of the healers has not yet extended to this inner realm, except only rarely.

However from an altogether different area some eighty years after Jung's momentous discovery once again the medium of the skin has begun to edge itself into a more central rôle. This is in the field of 'biofeedback' a name which is curiously informative.

The system described by Brown[16] "is a curious mixture of startling simplicity and challenging complexity, which is deceptively straightforward". By using a simple device to convert the activity of the body system into a form which can be sensed, the subject can learn to recognise those bodily feelings he has when for example the temperature is raised (or lowered) or the heart is beating fast, (or slowly). As Brown[17] states "it is probably the most complex of all the discoveries about man's being, for it points at the greatest mystery of all: the ability of the mind to control its own, and the body's sickness and health".

This highly complex field involved mechanisms which are not yet understood for the whole area where the psyche meets the soma is dark, and exceedingly mysterious. Biofeedback itself includes all manner of inter-reactions between the higher and lower brain centres, all the intellectual and emotional aspects of both conscious and unconscious psyche. The point where matter and spirit touch and undergo an enantiodromia, is the central locus of the greatest mystery of the life process, indeed it is possibly the mystery of life itself.

Undoubtedly biofeedback has become very popular because it is instantly understood and the participation of the individual subject is vital. It is at base, a technique for training, but the inclusion of the participant is a major step. It has proved itself to be a tool of paramount importance as regards the organ of the skin. Possibly because as Brown[18] points out, "it is a very private process, but mostly because the skin, whose extraordinary communications ability is only now beginning to be recognised".[19] The skin is "a body system almost without parallel for its ability to reflect the mental and emotional life of the body".[20] She makes a further interesting comment concerning the reaction of the skin in biofeedback[21] in comparison with other organs. "In the latter, the monitors reveal information which appears to relate to changes within the systems themselves." Consequently the expression of the emotional and mind function tends to be a secondary consideration to the life supporting function. For example the heart beat as the prime expression of the physical health of the heart, and as the secondary expression of the emotional background of the individual. However with the organ of the skin, its electrical reactions do not express the skin's functions, or the skin's health as such, or indeed anything about the skin, on the contrary "the skin tells us about the mind".[22]

About one hundred years after the remarkable series of events described above which led to Jung's early discoveries, it is now relatively commonplace to speak of the unconscious. In retrospect it has become clear that the work processes described and involving many able minds represented a constellation of events which led to the establishment of the scientific birth of the unconscious mind. Man was to become consciously aware of the presence of the unconscious. It was the association test which drew Jung's attention to the complexes which are present in all human beings. A complex may be defined as an unconscious or half conscious aggregate of representations laden with emotion. It is a field of associations surrounding a central nucleus. One might also describe it as a psychic mirror or reflection, of a bodily cell, where the nucleus or the power house is surrounded by the cytoplasm which is its support system. A complex can be acquired by personal experience during the lifetime or its nucleus can be formed by an archetypal content. If the emotion should become either intense, or overwhelming it can lead to every kind of neurotic or pathological disturbance. In the word association test it was the emotion associated with the complexes which was revealed by the test words which related to it. This was the cause of the disturbances to which Jung applied his formidable intellect, with such momentous results.

The organ of the skin is the one bodily organ above all others which serves as the paramount psychic reflector; a crystalline mirror which permits the visualization of psychic disturbance in a singularly graphic form. The many and varied skin disease processes which beset the organ either of a transient or apparently permanent nature, provide an unique and in depth understanding of the psychic life of the individual concerned. They express underlying anxieties, hidden fears, unrecognised emotions of every hue, and indicate the unconscious psychic complex. The skin reflects, as does a mirror the unconscious psyche of man. It has always been the habitude of the physician to look through the skin at the underlying soma. Now it is the task of the dermatologist, and those interested in the skin, not to be satisfied solely with the dermatosis, but to look through the skin, at psyche.

Jung was to discover in his research that complexes are autonomous, possessing an innate driving force, and can be all powerful in controlling thoughts and behaviour. Such is their nature that a person does not have a complex, on the contrary, indeed, the complex has him. Furthermore complexes need not necessarily be an impediment to the adjustment to life of the subject. In fact it is often the contrary, inspiration and drive which are essential for achievement have their sources in the complexes.

The question which concerned Jung was how do complexes originate?

It was the vital question in Jung's researches, which eventually led him to the discovery of a very deep level where the complexes originated. This level is much deeper in human nature than the early experiences of childhood. This discovery brought to consciousness the whole vast world of objective psyche to which Jung was later to give the name of the collective unconscious. The answer therefore to his vital question concerning the origination of the complexes was the collective unconscious. This concept was later to be substantiated by Jung's immense researches into alchemy. This monumental work, on his part was of an extraordinary magnitude, and occupied him for many years. Alchemy had been practised for some seventeen hundred years, by scholars, physicians and priests, who usually worked in solitude. Their labours constellated round a central goal, which was ostensibly to transform base metals into gold, on one level. However they were also engaged in the great work of the search for the elixir of life or the philosophical stone of the wise. This was the lapis philosophorum, the stone of immortality. Alchemy was essentially a transformation process and did in fact, in the 17th century, transform itself into the science which was to become, eventually, modern chemistry. By so doing it ceased to exist as alchemy.

As has been seen nothing ever disappears, and so alchemy fell away into the unconscious where it remained for two hundred years. It was Jung's destiny to take up again this neglected discipline. He collected thousands of manuscripts of those ancient and forgotten men. He deciphered, and translated the Latin, Greek, Arabic, Mediaeval European and other texts. This was not an easy task, because the contents of the documents, were entirely alien to modern European consciousness.

In this vast treasure house of knowledge he discovered the historical substrata of the psyche of mankind and with it, the substantive proof for his concepts, which he had formulated with his own confrontation with the unconscious. He was thus able to distinguish and to prove the existence and the reality of this vast collective unconscious psychic realm, as a deeper stratum to that of the personal unconscious. This layer is composed of the eternal archetypes, which are in themselves impenetrable and unknowable. They are recognised by their images only. An archetype is a dynamism which always makes itself felt in the numinosity and fascinating power of its image. It can only be recognised therefore by the effect it produces. Jung said[23] "the archetype as an image of instinct is a spiritual goal towards which the whole of man strives". Jung's discovery of the collective unconscious psyche was of far greater significance than the discovery of the complex. It was eventually to establish his reputation as one of the outstanding intellects of this century.

With the formulation of this concept Jung was to reveal that as there was a master plan for the body, provided by evolution and heredity, so also was there an equivalent master plan for psyche. Until the advent of this concept psychology had been confined to the strictly environmental determinism of the mind. By means of this highly significant step, Jung was able to sunder the ties and free himself from the former views. There is no doubt that this discovery was a turning point in the history of psychology since it was an event of the utmost magnitude. Moreover he confirmed the view held by Carus[24] "the key to an understanding of the nature of the conscious life of the soul lies in the sphere of the unconscious". Jung was thus able to bring to consciousness the vastness of the psyche as a whole whilst at the same time, he was able to define and bring into perspective ego's fundamental importance and also its limitations against this dark and immense background.

In a time span of a century, after centuries of enquiry the concept of the unconscious psyche was realized and eventually established by these physicians.

Although this vital realization has been made available to all, it has not yet been integrated into consciousness by the medical profession in general. Consequently the tremendous significance of its rôle in the aetiology of all somatic disease remains outside medical consciousness, to its grave and indeed certain loss. The reasons for this collective non-acceptance lies primarily in the fact that ideas of such immensity are not easy to assimilate quickly by the rational intellect. After all one cannot see, hear, taste, touch, or feel the unconscious realm as is the case with the reality world. A century is as nothing compared to the history of objective psyche which is millions of years old. In the academic medical world, the goal of medical thought is directed towards problem solution in a pragmatic and practical manner. Such inductive thinking constitutes the essential of medical learning. This has led to a singular brand of modern medical materialism, especially geared to the technological advancements inherent in the modern world. This type of thinking has a particular adamantine brilliance which is seductively attractive by the fact that it appears to cast few shadows, but it is curiously hard, lacking in empathy and human warmth. Such minds so attuned, find it exceedingly difficult if not impossible to encompass another world, other than the reality world of our existence. Confronted by this other realm, fear is engendered, and an aggressively fortified resistance develops.

Ego consciousness has undoubtedly and wisely so to speak erected and strengthened its ramparts against the slow rhythmic tide of unconscious currents. It is not for everyone, fortunately, to encounter this unknown territory, but for some it is vital for health that they should realize its objective nature. These are those who suffer, from whatever illness, be it somatic or psychic. All must confront the inner reality and it behoves the physician to learn something of its existence and also of his own nature.

REFERENCES

1 Rook, A. Wilkinson, D.S. Ebling, F. J. Textbook of Dermatology, Third Edition, 1979, Blackwell.
2 Jung, C. G., C. G. Jung Letters, Vol. 2., p.4.
3 Ibid., Vol. 1., p.119
4 Jung, C. G., Collected Works, Vol. 2, para 1036 Psychophysical Investigations with the Galvanometer, and Pneumograph in Normal and Insane Individuals.
5 Peterson, F. & Jung, C. G. Brain: A Journal of Neurology (London) XXX (1907), 118 (July), p.153-218
6 Tarcharoff, J. Pflug. Arch. ges Physiol XLV1 (1890), 46–55.
7 Galton, I Francis, "Psychometric Experiments", Brain II (1897), 149–62.
8 Wündt, Wilhelm, In Wündt Philosophische Studien X 1892 326–28
9 Kraepelin, Emil "Experimentelle Studien über Assoziationen", Freiburg 1883
10 Aschaffenburg, Gustav, Psychol. Arb.I (1896) 209-99II (1899) 1–82IV (1904), 253-374.
11 Sommer, Robert and Fürstenau, Robert Halle I (1906): 3, 197-207.
12 Muller, E. K., Verhandlung LXXXVII (1904), 79-80 (summary of paper read 1 August 1904 to Section for Medicine)
13 Veraguth, OttoArch.psychol. VI (1907), p.162-163.
14 Jung, C. G., Collected Works, Vol.2 para 1042-1043
15 Hannah, Barbara, Jung his Life and Work A biographical memoir, Putnam 1976, p.80
16 Brown, B. B Ph.D. Introduction. New Mind New Body, Harper & Row, July 1984.
17 Ibid.
18 Ibid.
19 Ibid.
20 Ibid.
21 Ibid. (Chapter 2)
22 Ibid.
23 Jung, C. G., Collected Works Vol. 8. para 415 2nd Edition Routledge & Kegan Paul, London.
24 Carus, Carl Gustav, Psyche, 1846, On the Development Of the Soul, Introduction, p.1, Spring Publications, 1970, New York City.

PART I

THE SKIN AS SYMBOL OF
TRANSFORMATION AND REBIRTH

For untold thousands of years, animal skins of the reptilian avian and mammalian species have taken precedence over all other bodily organs as objects of reverential awe.

In order to discover as to why this has been so, in the past and still today amongst primitive peoples, it may be helpful to examine what men have thought felt sensed and imagined about this most singular of organs.

It is not unusual in the dreams of modern man for human figures to appear covered in fish scales or feathers or with the skin of an animal such as the horse dog cat or even a bear. Sometime even the wings of a bird.

Therefore the mythology attached to the organ of the skin must be considered carefully and in depth, as it is of immense importance for those who wish to understand the symbolic language of the unconscious psyche of mankind.

SKIN AND HIDE
(A BRIEF ETYMOLOGICAL STUDY)

The organ of the skin is the continuous flexible integument forming the usual external covering of the body of a human being, or of other animal bodies. The word is also used when describing one or other of the separate layers of which the integument is composed, the derma or the epidermis. In the English language the same word skin is also applied to the integument of an animal, stripped from the body and dressed or tanned with or without hair, or intended for this purpose, a hide pelt or fur. The same word describes the complete hide of a sheep such as sheepskin. Parchment or vellum used for writing is described as skin, since it is specially prepared from animal hides such as those obtained from calves or sheep. In the Icelandic language parchment or manuscripts are said to be 'skinns'.

The word skin has been in the English language since the thirteenth century. There has been a wide variation of the spelling. The word itself is derived from the old Norman word 'skinne' – which gave rise to skinn, skyn, and skiyn, later, sckyn, and skynn gave way to skynne, again in the 16th century.

The above spellings are closely connected with the Nordic skinn, Old High German scindan, and the German schinden. But the modern German word for skin is 'haut' closely allied to the Dutch 'huid' and the English word hide, for a dressed animal skin.

In France, the word for skin is peau, derived from an ancient twelfth century word pel, which stems from the Latin word for skin pellis, related to the Spanish language piel Portugese pele, and Italian pelle. The English word pelt is that given to an animal's skin and has the same derivation. Likewise in German, the word pelz is an animal's skin whilst the word in the Dutch language is vels.

The modern English language word dermis, is derived from the Greek word for skin, *derma*. Two other Greek words in common usage are corium, xopiov, which means skin or leather, and psora, which means scaly. The former corium, is the outermost layer enveloping the foetus at birth, and the modern anatomical definition today is the cutis vera which means the true skin. The latter psora, has been used in the English language since the late seventeenth century. It is the name applied to the ubiquitous dermatosis – psoriasis. The word saurian is now attached to the reptilian species, i.e. the lizard and the snake.

In general parlance the earth's crust may be described as a skin as is the iron plating of a vessel, the rind of certain fruits, or the bark of a tree. In all of these it means the façade, the outer limitation of the object's phenomenal existence, but also its protection of the individual's inner being.

Again generally speaking in certain phrases 'skin' is used to denote severe treatment, such as 'skinned', denoting theft of money by open robbery, or by stealth or by being cheated. In such cases the victim is described as being 'skinned'. Sometimes severe emaciation by starvation or illness is described as 'skin and bone'. An escape from catastrophe is described as 'to sleep in a whole skin'. One may be said to be 'out of one's skin' denoting extreme emotion, high spirits, fear, delight or shock. The Biblical Job said he had escaped with the skin of his teeth, when he survived, at last, the severe and unjust trials sent by God.

In these phrases, identification with the skin is observed, and in some instances with life itself. The idea is supported that the skin serves as the boundary of ego-personality as well as its protection, and defence.

The conclusion is unmistakable, the skin is a mediator between consciousness and the reality world on the one hand, and with the inner unconscious personality on the other.

Finally when skin is used as a verb it has a number of meanings, to cover, clothe, attire, all having a positive connotation, whereas to strip, deprive, flay or peel, as well as rub scrape or bark indicates depletion. The strange word 'skinbound' is rarely used but hidebound is frequently, to describe a person of fixed ideas rigidity of thought or ways of behaviour in those who are unable to adapt to the new.

1

THE RÔLE OF THE SKIN
IN MYTHOLOGY

In the history of mankind the cult of the animal with its sacrifice, has a long tradition.

Early in the last century, the eminent Swiss physician who became the founder of analytical psychology Carl Gustav Jung[1] in a letter to Sigmund Freud, wrote of the animal cult as practised by primitive man. "It is explained by an infinitely long psychological development which is of paramount importance and not by primitive bestial tendencies. These are nothing but the quality that provides the material for building a temple. But the temple and its meaning have nothing whatever to do with the quality of the building stones."

What then did the animal cults and their animal sacrifices signify?

The ritual sacrifices were made on certain feast days devoted to a particular god. Naturally they were originally connected with food as a gift for the god and also for the dead. In the course of the sacrificial rite, the skin of the animal was removed by flaying and conserved, but the flesh was eaten by the believers or participants. The skin was preserved, because it was believed to be sacred. This led millennia ago to reverential treatment of the animal skin as a cult object.

These practices were universal, and many animals were involved in cultic practice in diverse areas of the ancient world. However two animals in particular have been chosen for a closer study of such practice, in which the skin of the animal plays a pivotal rôle. One is the bear, which represents the prehistoric Northern Hemisphere of our world, and the other is the ram, as representative of the Ancient Mediterranean world in the pre-Christian era.

I. THE SKIN OF THE BEAR

A modern European is unlikely to conjecture as to how such cities as Berlin and Berne arrived at their particular names. Few would be interested even to know that the name benefactor is the bear. Nowadays the bear in general can only be seen in dreams, or pacing restlessly in a city zoo, or dispiritedly performing undignified acts in a travelling circus.

Today, only by good fortune a glimpse may be obtained of a solitary animal upon a mountain top, in the ice fields of Siberia, or in a protected forest reserve. But alas nowhere else, for the bear has all but vanished, but in pre-history he was believed to be, and was worshipped as a divinity.

Only in the vast underground sulphurous caverns below the surface of Europe in the transalpine regions can emanations of the mysterious breath of bears be perceived, or by the light of a flickering torch the scratch marks of their long dead claws may still be observed in the bitterly cold darkness of these forgotten places. The sombre mists of time have obscured the knowledge that amongst all those ancestral primitive peoples of Europe, Northern Euro-Asia, the North American continent, and the Circumpolar regions, the bear was treated with great respect. His terrifying strength, and his cunning were greatly feared, his enormous intelligence was regarded with awe, and reverence. But over and above this the bear was regarded as a god, and worshipped as such, because of his divine powers. He was thought to be at times masculine, at others, a feminine animal. However he was in a way a messenger of the gods, a hermetic figure appearing as the spirit of those vast, seemingly indestructible forests. As such he was therefore essentially a feminine animal, representing the earth itself. The centuries passed but even in the epoch of the Celts, the tribal forefathers of the European races, the breath of sanctity still clung to the bear. He represented the spirit of the warrior class, nobility above all, strength courage and cunning, all qualities possessed by the Celts themselves. The bear was undoubtedly the worthy recipient, as a bearer of these qualities of their unconscious projections,

Briefly it is well to recall that the word bear in the Celtic language was 'Artos' closely related to the Irish 'art' and the Gaulish 'arth', and from which incidentally the modern masculine name of 'Arthur' is derived.

Little is known of the nature of religion in those early Palaeolithic and Neolithic civilizations. However it can safely be said that in the former civilization its people were hunters, whilst in the latter, and the Bronze age, agricultural or pastoral life was essential to the life of man. As such, animal gods were the great deities.

It is clear that in the past although bear worship was ubiquitous not a great deal was known of it amongst primitive peoples until about forty years or so ago. Considerable research by Japanese and Russian scientists has been undertaken amongst many primitive peoples in the circumpolar region. They are the Altaic peoples, the Tungu and the Yakuts of Siberia. A wealth of information is gradually being prepared for general dissemination. The Yakuts, in speaking of the bear say today, 'he hears all, recalls all, and forgets nothing'. However it is the Aino, (or Ainu) of the northern part of the Japanese archipelago, the Keril islands, and Hokkaido where the information gleaned is singularly helpful. The Aino of these areas are also found in the U. S. S. R. at Yuzho (Yesa) and Sakhalin island (Saghalien).

Frazer[2] says, the "Ainu worshipped the bear after their fashion". For them, the bear provided food from its flesh, and its skin provided the means to pay tributes or taxes, and supplied clothing. Many varieties of a legend have been handed down, that a woman of the Ainu had a child from a bear, and many mountain peoples pride themselves on being descended from a bear. This is an example of the bear-son motif. In Japanese, the term is Kamui Sanikiri – Descendants of the Bear. An individual will say he is descended from the divine one which rules in the mountains, meaning the 'god of the mountains' no other than the bear.

Throughout this whole region of the Ainu bear festivals were held, and the central idea was the ritual sacrifice of the bear. A young bear cub was brought up carefully with protection and good nourishment until it reached adult status and had waxed fat. Then it was killed and afterwards flayed. Before the sacrificial killing, the Aino of Yuzho issued an invitation to the feast, in order, "to unite in great pleasure to send the god away". Then followed a lengthy speech made to the bear to remind him that he had been protected and nourished and now he must be killed. He was then exhorted to speak well of his captors when he met his father and mother in the land of his ancestors. Other prayers in the same vein, showed clearly that the bear was regarded as both god, and spirit messenger. The Aino of Sakhalin also pleaded with the bear that he would request the gods to supply his benefactors with rare furs (the skin of animals) and animals good to eat, fish in the seas, and seals on the shores. Then followed a final request that the bear would overcome all those spirits evilly disposed towards man. At last he was despatched, so that he would be able to accomplish these requested benefactions.

However running like a thread through all these ceremonial rituals, there is a singular emphasis upon the skin of the bear. It was usually and eventually traded for material benefits, but after flaying, the conserved skin together with the skull, was treated with reverence, in that it was always carried into the central place of honour, so that he (the bear) could watch over all the post-sacrificial aspects of the ceremony.

The flayed skin of the bear did not just represent the dead bear – it was the soul of the bear.

Furthermore it was never permitted to cross the threshold of the central dwelling where the ritual feast took place, but had to be taken down the smoke hole or through a window if present. The bear's skin at all times

was treated with exquisite reverence, and throughout the presiding ceremonial it was exactly as if the living bear was participating in the subsequent feasting.

Undoubtedly these facts point to the inescapable conclusion that the bear
skin itself was regarded as divine. Interestingly enough the bear feasts
always took place in the autumn after the bear had been fed on the abundant food in the summer. The tribes in their turn feasted upon the bear,
reserving the pelt for both physical and spiritual blessings to come.

THE SKIN OF THE RAM
I EGYPT.

The ram along with other horned animals the male goat, the stag and the
bull embodied fertility. Solar gods were linked always with the heavenly
ram, Aries.

In Ancient Egypt the ram Khnemu was worshipped, as one of the most
ancient of all the gods of Egypt. Khnemu is connected with the root Khnem
which means to join, to unite or to build.[3] Khnemu was worshipped at Her-
akleopolis, Elephantine, and at Esna as well as at other places, including
Mendes where he was worshipped as a local animal god.

The word for soul in Egypt was Ba and as the name for ram was also
Ba, the title Ba-neb-Tettu was sometimes held to mean, 'the soul, the Lord
Tettu'. This was the local form of Khnemu, whose symbol there at Mendes
was the ram, as elsewhere.[4]

At Elephantine, Khnemu was regarded as the source and the guardian of
the Nile, as he brought forth the floods. He was primarily a creator god
who fashioned a child on a potter's wheel and implanted him as a seed in
his mother's body. He also made the gods, and was the father of fathers,
and the mother of mothers. He also assisted at the birth of all things. He
was, "Ram as the virile male, the holy phallus which stirreth up the passions of love, the Ram of rams, whose gifts are brought forth by the earth,
after it has been flooded by the Nile, the soul, the life of Ra" (the sun).[5]

With its curved horns, the ram was the sacred animal of Amen who was
worshipped as a primeval god, but later as the great god of Thebes, circa
2133–1780 B. C. He was regarded as "the hidden one" for he was the effective force in the invisible wind. He was identified with the sun god, as
Amen-Ra, and became the god who abides in all things – thus he was the
'ba' or soul of all phenomena. Not only was the god himself said to be 'hidden' but his form or his similitude was 'unknown'. Applied to the great god
Amen, 'hidden' implied something more than the "sun which disappeared
below the horizon". It implied the god who cannot be seen by mortal eyes
the god who is both invisible and inscrutable to gods as well as to men.
One of the attributes applied to him was eternal.[6] Since the ram was the

divine animal, by the same token the attribute of eternal also applied to it.

At the end of the New Kingdom in Egypt, circa 1507–1320 B.C., animal cult centres sprang up. This was about the same time that the Book of the Dead was placed in the tombs. Certain animals were revered, the cat at Bubassus, the bull at Memphis, and the Ibis at Hermopolis. Since the animals as manifestations of the gods were protected, they were also revered as gods themselves. Thus they were enthroned, mummified after death, and interned.

The animals were the media of revelation and carriers of transcendental powers. The fact remains, the individual animal was the physical aspect of the transcendent image, the theriomorphic form of which expressed a particular aspect of divinity.

Sacred animals were therefore the ba, of the gods that is the eternal soul as we have seen with the ram. As with the bear, on feast days the sacrificial animal was flayed, the skin preserved and the flesh eaten. The flesh provided the nourishment, but again the skin as the soul of the god was the vehicle of the divine essence and treated with reverential awe.

However in this period, the animal skins were an important essentiality for the outer appearance during the achievement of a final inner transformation, the skin thus was the symbol of the transitional state.

In Egypt the skin had a central rôle in the ancient religion. The protector god of childbirth, Bes wore a lion skin, on his back. But later a panther skin was depicted on his breast. Three fox skins served as a written sign for birth.

The long and difficult, highly skilled techniques performed in the embalming process of the funerary rites of Ancient Egypt were accompanied by a complicated ceremony with prayers readings and incantations. The final part of this long and particularly precise ceremony was the 'opening of the mouth'[7] in which the panther animal skin worn by the Sem priest played a central rôle. The actual mummification process aimed at, and succeeded in, preserving the body of the defunct, but particular emphasis was made to establish preservation of the skin. Undoubtedly the place accorded to the animal skin worn by the priest had operated in this fashion during the course of many centuries.

The skin of the panther, as an agent of transformation in itself, served to bestow a complete and absolute divinity upon the wearer who then became the god, with the power to transform the deceased into immortality. As the skin appeared to be imperishable and indestructible it was therefore regarded as being eternal.

Thus the skin of the animal carried the soul of the animal, and since the animal is divine, so was the skin divine. This indispensable accompaniment was it seems, the vital link in the mummification whereby the defunct became the god Osiris – thus divine, and eternal.

In the same book the Book of the Dead there is another ceremony in the

Judgement of the defunct. It is called the 'Weighing of the Heart of the Dead'[8]. The defunct is led into the prescence of Osiris, the god of the dead, enthroned within a shrine in the form of a funerary chest. Before him is a lotus flower near which hangs the skin of an animal. The lotus belongs to the god Nefertem described as a lotus bloom with the nose of Ra the sun god. Therefore he is a god of fragrance and a solar divinity. As such he is associated with rebirth.

Again, the idea of rebirth is connected in the Egyptian religion, with the mysterious Tekenu. Earlier representations show it to be a crouching man wrapped in skin from head to toe. In later representations the Tekenu consisted of a pear-shaped bundle of a naked man with arms and legs drawn in. The Tekenu was a ceremonial object which appeared to have had its origin in extremely archaic burial cultures which included such attributes of archaic burial as the animal skin wrap and the crouching position. This foetal position is very widespread and a common feature of archaic burial.

Lurker,[9] says "The significance attached to the Tekenu is not clear. It has been thought to be a symbolic representation of human sacrifice by some, whereas others see it as a substitute image of the deceased as a kind of scapegoat to confront the uncanny powers of the next world".

The notion of rebirth was presumably concerned with the skin under which the Tekenu lay in the crouching position. Most probably it represented a transitional stage onwards towards rebirth. A substantive and relatively modern report from the early years of this century informs of a King of the Shankalla tribe of Ethiopia who was sewn up in a green hide bag in a sitting position prior to burial.

Jung[10] in a letter to Michaelis in writing of the psychology of Ancient Egypt in the millennia before the Christian era says "On one side a torpid impersonal unconscious reigned, on the other a revealed consciousness, or a consciousness inspired from within and hence derived directly from the gods, personified in Pharoah".

He was the Self, and the individual of the people. The spirit still came from above. The tension between above and below was undoubtedly extreme, hence the opposites held together only by means of equally rigid forms". He continues[11]

> "the tension between the above and the below in Ancient Egypt . . . is the real source of Near Eastern saviour figures, whose patriarch is Osiris. He is also the source of the idea of an individual (immortal) soul. The purpose of nearly all rebirth rites is to unite the above with the below. The baptism in Jordan is an eloquent example, water below Holy Ghost above."

On the primitive level, the totemistic rite of renewal is always a reversion to the half-animal, half-human condition of pre-historic times. Hence the frequent use of animal skins and other animal attributes. Evidence of this is found in the cave paintings discovered in the South of France. Among these customs, we must reckon the demotion of high to low. In Christianity the washing of the disciples' feet, in Ancient Egypt the birth from an animal's skin."

In these examples examined it is clearly evident that there was an immense mana attached to the skin and for these ancient peoples was equivalent to the immortal eternal soul.

II THE SKIN OF THE RAM IN GREECE.

1. Zeus

In his report of the great festival of Zeus in Thebes, in Greece, Herodotus[12] describesthe legend in which Zeus, the mighty Zeus appears in a ram's skin, holding the head of the ram before him.

The Thebans came to regard the ram as a holy animal and sacrificed it at the festival of Zeus once year. On this day the ram was flayed after sacrifice and its skin used to cover the image of Zeus. Amidst lamentation the ram was then buried in a sacred tomb, as the essence or divinity of the god.

2. The Golden Fleece

The sanctity with which the ram was held in the Bronze Age in the Aegean is revealed in the beautiful legend of Helle and Phrixos. These were the children of King Athamas, whose second wife wanted to murder them. Their mother Nephele rescued them by placing them on the golden ram supplied by Hermes, the god who is most helpful and obliging in times of abject helplessness. The ram which was the colour of the beautiful gold of the sun, carried the children across the straits dividing Asia from Europe. Alas Helle, the little girl fell in and was drowned, but Phrixos, her brother landed safely and immediately sacrificed the golden ram to Zeus, in thanksgiving for his life.

He then gave the golden fleece to King Aetes in exchange for one of his daughters. In turn, the King consigned the precious golden fleece to the care of a monstrous dragon, who became from that moment the guardian of this great treasure. Eventually the miraculous fleece became the coveted goal of Jason and the Argos expedition.

The perilous quest became the synonym[13] for "attaining the unobtainable. The golden fleece unites the two symbols, the innocence of the ram, and the glory of the gold. The dragon killed heroically is the symbol of the real liberation."

The Horned Gods

During the Bronze and Iron Ages, horned deities were found in Europe, the Near and Middle East, and also Egypt and India. The horns signified divinity. The chief of the horned gods of Egypt, as has been seen, was Amon.

Evidence from the painted and sculpted caves in Europe has revealed that Paleolithic and Neolithic man possessed certain religious or magical ceremonials in which a horned man, presumably a god, took the central place. The now well-known drawing of a stag-horned man in the Caverne des Trois Frères in Ariège in France represents the most important of the horned figures of the late Paleolithic period amongst the effigies and drawings of this mysterious horned figure. It is difficult in the cave to find the drawing as it is in an obscure part of the cavern, but when found it engenders in the observer a distinct numinosum singularly perceived by those who are fortunate to be able to view it. It has to be said that the period when human hands made this drawing, is so far removed from modern consciousness that it is impossible to know the real meaning embodied.

The figure which appears to be that of a man is clothed in the skin of a stag, and is wearing the stag's antlers. The hide of the animal covers the whole of the man's body, the hands and feet being drawn as if seen through a transparent gauze. The eyes are startling, being large round set in a bearded face, and intensely alive. Many who have seen the figure, describe the gaze as piercing. The appearance is undoubtedly that of a human being.

He is holding a musical intrument possibly a flute or a pipe, and is surrounded by animals. It is generally agreed that he is performing a ceremonial dance, or a ritualized movement. This ancient drawing reveals that the hide is of a stag and it is evident that the human figure in the light of other comparative religions is a shaman, who in donning the animal skin[14] "assumes the numinous powers assigned to deity", and so he himself becomes and is indeed then the god. A similar Bronze-Age figure found at Mojenjo-Daro in India, also clothed in a hairy animal skin probably that of a bull, with bull horns, and surrounded by animals is known as Pasupati, a form of Shiva as Lord of the Animals. The similarity, of this figure to that of the Ariège figure is so pronounced that one may assume an equivalence of meaning.

Since antiquity, the belief that the gods revealed themselves in dreams and declared their will to mankind was widespread. This led as is well known, to temple pilgrimages to seek blessing or healing spiritually and physically.

Livy[15] in describing such, informs of a ritual in Attica, where the skin of a sacrificed ram was flayed. The pilgrim suppliant to the temple then slept upon it, until he received a revelation from the god in a dream. The flayed hide as the immortal soul of the god permitted access to the god's benevolence during the time of transition.

In the comparatively recent past, in various parts of East Africa the skin

35

of a sacrificed ram or a goat was cut into strips and placed round the wrists of those who were ill or needed protection against disease. The same ritual applied to newly born children, as it is a common belief still in parts of Africa that ill-luck often attached itself to the newly-born.

A strange ceremony 'the being born again', or 'born of a goat' is observed even today amongst the children of the Kikuya. The ritual[16] proceeded when the child concerned was ten or eleven years. A circular piece of skin from a sacrificed goat was passed over one shoulder and under the other of the child to be born again. The mother of the child or a woman who acted as mother, sat on a hide of a goat on the floor, with the child between her knees.

Then the goat or ram's gut was passed over her and brought in front of the child. The woman then groaned as if in labour and then she cut the animal's gut just as if it was the umbilical cord. The child then imitated the cry of a new born baby. This ceremony used to be combined with that of circumcision but later this practice was divided into two different rites. All over the horn of Africa this ceremony is still practised in the remoter areas.

The rebirth is in effect a spiritual rebirth with the concomitant sacrifice of attachment to the mother, on the human emotional level. Again the rôle of the animal skin is central in the transition.

In other parts of East Africa, again goats were sacrificed, and the skin was used to cure skin diseases of the hands. The same practice was observed by the Masai in the Masai Mara in Kenya. Again a sacrificial goat skin was used to preserve the health of man. All participants at these ceremonies wore rings made from animal skin which served as amulets against disease and ill-luck. Flaying of the animals served as a potent protection against evil spirits.

All of these rites and tribal practices clearly show there was an exceedingly archaic and ubiquitous belief that the skin embodied deity, which accounted for its immense mana everywhere.

Finally on this same note, the Issapoo tribe from the island of Fernando Po[17] in West Africa regard the cobra as their guardian deity. Every year a cobra was ritually killed in a special ceremonial, and the skin preserved with meticulous care.

The flayed snake's skin was fastened to a branch of the tallest tree in the village, by the head, with the tail hanging down.

After subsequent acts of ceremonial all the children born during the previous year were carried to the hanging serpent skin, and their hands were placed on its tail. The skin of the totem animal as the soul of the tribal god, brought protection for the child against ill-luck. It was an act of propriation since the guardian deity was believed either to bestow good or ill- luck. Clearly the animal skin was treated with the greatest reverence far and wide in the old world since time immemorial. But what of the New World? An answer may be sought in central America.

THE RÔLE OF HUMAN SKIN IN MEXICAN MYTHOLOGY.

It has been seen that an individual may assume the characteristics of the totem animal by donning the skin of that animal. There is an analogy with the sacrificial rites practised by the priests of pre-Columbian Mexico. Of all the Mexican vegetation deities the most important, and the most terrifying by far, was Xipe-Totec[18] (Our Lord the Flayed).

He was always represented as clad in a human skin stripped from the body of a sacrificial captive.

Xipe-Totec as the god of renewal and vegetation represented the fresh skin which the Earth receives from the recurrent green in the Springtime. Therefore the great festival which was called, the 'Feast of the Man-Flaying' was always held at the time of the Spring equinox,when the fresh verdure first appeared in that dry and barren land. In the eyes of the people, the actual greening was miraculous, and believed to be the actual prescence of the god.

At these festivals, captive human beings were sacrificed, these included men women and children. After being killed, they were flayed, the skins were conserved. and then worn by the personators of the god. The captor however of an individual victim did not eat the particular flesh of his own captive because he regarded it as part of his own body. He himself as sacrificer, became the sacrificed one.

The essence of the festival[19] was strange, in that a prisoner of war was taken, the most gallant whom they had at hand and a ceremony of testing was performed upon him. He was fastened by a rope to the central hole of a stone of flat cylindrical shape, the so-called temalacatl. (Spinning wheel of stone.) Eventually after defending himself to the point of exhaustion he was shot with arrows so that his blood would drop and fertilize the earth. This was the original form of the ceremony, but in Mexico City, the exhausted prisoner was sacrificed by cutting open the breast, and tearing out the heart. Many prisoners were sacrificed after him, and their skins were flayed and donned as described.

The human sacrifice was absolutely vital in the course of religious process. The flayed skins were believed to be possessed of a power of enchantment and were thus regarded with reverence. The magic properties imbued in the skins were invoked by the wearing of the skin for twenty-one daysby all those who were afflicted with eye or skin diseases. The three week cycle is interesting, Xipe-Totec was originally a very ancient moon god, and planting of crops generally in those far off days took place at certain periods of the moon cycle. Today in the discipline of dermatology, the average number of days for epidermal cell turnover is about twenty-one days.

Xipe-Totec's colour was yellow his ornaments golden, but he always was clad in a green garment, symbolic of the green grain, the maize as it first appeared before it ripened to deepest gold. The god because of the associated gold colour was the patron of the gold workers because it was believed that the gold came out of the earth, like the maize.

At this festival, which included dancing a hymn was sung, the following is one which has been preserved, and was sung by the young warriors, and the observers.

Hymn to Xipe-Totec[20]

"Thou night time drinker, why does thou delay?
Put on thy disguise, thy golden garment put it on,
My Lord, let thy emerald waters, come descending
Now is the old tree changed to green plumage
The Fire Snake is transformed into the Quetzal
If may be that I am to die, I the young maize plant
Like an emerald in my heart; gold would I see it be;
I shall be happy when first it is ripe – the war chief is born.
My Lord, when there is abundance in the maize fields,
I shall look to thy mountains, verily thy worshipper,
I shall be happy when first it is ripe – the war chief is born."

The transformation of the fire snake into the Quetzal, the wind god refers to the material change in the maize crop occasioned by the advent of the winds, the forerunners of the blessed rains.

The mock battle always encapsulated into the Xipe-Totec ceremonial festival was conducted by the young men, and signified an initiation of the young immature youths into manhood and the warrior class.

The rôle of the human skin is central in the entire drama, as initiator, transforming agent, and also as healing factor. When worn by the youths, its rôle as vehicle of the deity transferred its divine nature upon the wearer. The young men thus became the maize god, and were maize shoots and like the grain itself, had to transform from youth into maturity and sacrifice. The skin was the undoubted numinous transforming agent.

The reference to the war chief harks back to the war god Huitzilo puchtli the Humming Bird of the South or god of the Southern sun, whose attribute was the fire-serpent. He was also the national deity of the ruling tribe of the Aztec nation, and dreadfully feared because of searing drought which came in the wake of the summer land winds. This god was the child of the earth goddess Coatlicue "She of the serpent woven skirts" one of the most abjectly terrifying of all goddesses.

As one steps through the barren land of Mexico with its carpet of serpents one can feel her prescence and realize the innate meaning everywhere.

The priests of Xipe-Totec, and the young men chosen for the mock battle of the festival, were all clad in the human skins flayed from the sacrificial victims, in like manner to the god himself. The idea seemed to be that as the god is placated with human blood, in order to secure the generation and maturity of the grain, so it is with youth of the nation, who must grow like the maize towards maturity in the golden flowering of the young warriors, with the eventual probability of sacrifice, like the grain itself.

MAN FLAYING BY THE FINGER CUTTERS OF ALBANIA.

Some fifteen hundred years ago in the early centuries of Christianity, Moses of Kalankata[21] the Armenian historian wrote of the activities of the finger cutters in the 5th century A.D.

This sect had apparently, an affinity with devil worship and witchcraft. Vatchaken, the King of Albania at the time was a zealous persecutor of all heathen practices, and had the finger cutters placed firmly in his sights. Whilst this task was undertaken, a boy came to his notice who reported that he had seen the body of a young man pegged out on the ground, and stretched by the thumbs and great toes. Then whilst the young man on the ground was still alive he was flayed.

The witness was espied and chased but managed to escape by hiding from the finger cutters, and was able thus to observe the entire ritual. The participants were arrested and put to torture, but no confession was evinced. Execution was ordered and as they were led off, the King singled out one of the young men, and through promise of life and freedom, he was induced to confess the entire procedure of these secret gatherings.

The young man who confessed gave a strange testimony. He said:

"The devil comes in the form of a man and commands people to stand in three groups. One group holds the victim, and without wounding or slaying him, the whole skin is taken off along with the thumb of the right hand and carried across the chest to the little finger of the left hand, which is also cut off and taken along. The same process is repeated on the feet, whilst the victim is still alive. Thereupon he is put to death, the skin is then freed from the body, prepared, and laid in a basket.

When the time of the evil worship arrives they make or set up a folding chair of iron with feet, which closely resemble the feet of that man (or the feet of man?). They place the previous garment on the chair. The devil comes, puts on this garment, and sits on the chair, and having taken the skin of the human sacrifice, along with the fingers, he is seen (becomes visible?) If they are unable to bring the customary tribute (of a human skin) he commands them to peel off the bark of a tree (= the skin of the tree). They also sacrifice before him cattle and sheep, whose flesh he partakes in the company of his wicked ministers. (Further) they saddle a horse, then he rides off until the horse stops. There he vanishes. This he does once a year."

Apparently after this confession the King's command was that all the prisoners should be in their turn flayed alive.

Writing in the fifth century A.D. Faustus of Byzantium[22] says of the imperfectly Christianized Armenia of the preceding century that they continued "in secret to worship the old deities in the form of fornication". This remark probably arose because of the sacred prostitution practised at the great and renowned sanctuary to the goddess Anahit, or Anaitis which were the Persian and Armenian names for Venus the Star of Ishtar and Astarte. The sanctuary was at Erez.

The Mithraic mysteries, though strongly masculine-orientated retained Anahit or Anahita as the female deity of creation.[23]

In all probability the ceremony so described, purported to be associated with witchcraft was perhaps a secret enactment of an ancient ceremonial involving human sacrifice to old gods of the ancient country of Albania situated in the Caucasus between the Black and Caspian seas, and under the dominion of the Parthian empire.

It may be recalled that the Armenian god, popular before the Christian era was Mihr (Parthian or Sassannian) for Mithra. He was believed to be a brother of the goddess Anahit. For the Armenians he was the fire god and was identified with Hephaistus in syncretistic times. The main fire festival of Armenia came always in February of the Armenian calendar.

Little is known of this god, butthe connection of Mihr with fire in Armenia may be explained as a result of an early identification with the native Vahagn, the sun lightning and fire god, the eighth god of the Armenian pantheon.

Vahagn as a fierce storm god who as in Vedic and Teutonic religions had supplanted the god of the bright heaven. It is possible that Vahagn may have once required human sacrifices in Armenia, as his Teutonic brother Wotan did.

A strange legend which may be connected with the finger cutters is that in the region of Sassun a legendary hero called Mehr was supposed to live with his horse as a captive in a cave which could, it seems, only be entered on Ascension night. There it is believed, he lived on, and turned constantly a wheel of fortune and will appear again at the end of the world – so prophecy has it.

The curious name of the sect, 'the finger cutters' also calls to mind the very ancient cult of Samothrace and Phrygia, characterised by the earth mother and her companions the Kabiri or dactyloi. These dwarves wore little hooded cloaks, implying invisibility. They were conceived as deities and since the dactyls are fingers, it is perhaps not inappropriate to allow assumption that the sect in question was also worshipping an archaic pagan feminine earth spirit, and her accompanying sun – the archaic native Vahagn, who preceded Mihr, long before Armenia was Christianized. The Kabiri represent creative impulses. Undoubtedly these ancient cults although ousted by the advent of Christianity lived on in the collective psyche of mankind. Indeed as do they still today, which accounts for the appearance even of Kabiri in the dreams of modern man.

At that period, in the early centuries of our era, the old cults would still be possessed of a strong dynamism in the collective psyche, particularly in the wilder and more remote areas such as Northern Armenia, and contiguous Albania. As Christianity achieved supremacy, and became firmly established fierce opposition would have been engendered, between the more advanced Christianized educated class and the general populace, always the last to be converted, but still bound by pagan practices.

Prosecution was inevitable, and secrecy was therefore essential for fear of retribution. Only those initiated into the various forbidden cults may possibly have been aware, even if only superficially of the true nature of the strange ceremonial described by Moses of Kalankata. Christianity's eventual domination over all opposition led to abnegation of the cults themselves and any attached meaning would tend to fade with time. But it must be added, never to disappear entirely.

The Albanian story suggests that the coming of the new religion, with concomitant denigration, of old beliefs, former gods and mythological beings initiated a counter reaction in the unconscious by the free floating of consequently unused libido which no longer had a goal. One may postulate that the central rôle of the flayed human skin, with the marked emphasis on the fingers, particularly the creative phallic thumb, was the means by which the strivings of the unconscious (represented by the Kabiri and dactyloi as creative impulses) permitted the dark god to become visible. The Kabiri themselves had been in their own day mighty gods with an inherent darkness.

Psychologically this indicates an unconscious content urging towards the light of consciousness.

The great loss afforded to these pagan peoples by the institution of Christianity was the loss of contact with the natural world, and its wealth of instinctual knowledge. The deprivation created an unstable equilibrium, and the mushrooming of sectarian beliefs represented attempts by the unconscious to compensate this loss.

At about the fourth or fifth centuries after Christ there was already a schism between the light Christ image, and the dark devil. The latter had been banished allowing only the light god. Evil as such was denied and was considered a privatio boni. The impulses came from the small gods (dactyloi or fingers) which carried the unconscious realisation of the supreme sig-

41

nificance of the dark god or the problem of the principle of evil, which in reality has never been more important than at the present time in the history of the human race. A time, when it is clear, mankind becomes ever more distant from the unconscious instinctual realm.

If the problem is not accepted or realized in consciousness, then the human being is caught and perhaps possessed by evil and is unconscious of that possession. It is very interesting to note that in the Albanian story, the devil only becomes visible through the agency of the human skin.

Jung[24] has this to say concerning sacrifice. "The essential thing in the mythical drama is not the concreteness of the figures nor is it important what sort of animal is sacrificed or what sort of god it represents; what alone is important is that an act of sacrifice takes place, that a process of transformation is going on in the unconscious whose dynamism, whose contents, and whose subject are themselves unknown but become visible indirectly to the conscious mind by stimulating the imaginative material at its disposal, clothing themselves in it like the dancers who clothe themselves in the skins of animals, or the priests in the skins of their human victims."

In retrospect one is able to perceive through the mists of thousands and thousands of years the slow but autonomous and inexorable transformation of the unconscious whereby in the same slow measure of the passage of time man has come to consciousness of himself as man. The organ of the skin as the carrier of the essence of this transformation albeit unknown to human consciousness continues to be pivotal in the process of certain individuals, today.

A word must be interposed here concerning the process of flaying, which has played such a central rôle in both animal and human sacrifice. It has been the accompaniment of religious practices everywhere from time immemorial. It was conducted by the Scythians with scalpings, the Chinese, in the old Attic fertility rites, in Ancient Mexico as described, and elsewhere. The example in nature of this renewal of the god or goddess by flaying is to be observed in the serpent skin casting which occurs every year, in a natural way. Flaying signifies change from a previous state to a better one, hence renewal and rebirth. The transformed one becomes a new being. Like scalping, flaying and also dismemberment all belong to the birth and revelation of the inner man. They represent stations as it were, towards increased consciousness and an increasing awareness of wholeness.

REFERENCES

1 Jung, C. G., C. G. Jung Letters, Vol. 1, p. 26, Routledge & Kegan Paul, London.
2 Frazer, J. G., The Killing of the Divine Animal, The Golden Bough, Chapter LII

3 Budge, E. A. Wallis, The Gods of the Egyptians, Vol. 2, p. 50, Dover Publications Inc., NY, 1969.

4 Ibid., p. 64

5 Ibid.

6 Ibid., p. 2.

7 The Egyptian Book of the Dead, Ch. XXIII, Trans. by Budge, E. A. Wallis.

8 Ibid., The Judgement

9 Lurker, Manfred, The Gods and Symbols of Ancient Egypt, (English Language), Thames & Hudson, 1980.

10 Jung, C. G., Letters, Vol. l, para 259-260, Routledge & Kegan Paul, London.

11 Ibid., p. 260.

12 Herodotus, History II, p. 42

13 Jung, C. G., Collected Works, Vol. 12, para 206, Routledge & Kegan Paul, London.

14 Mead, M. A., The God of Witches, p. 24, Oxford Press.

15 Ibid.

16 Frazer, J. G., Folklore in The Old Testament, Part 2, Chapter3, Macmillan & Co.

17 Frazer, J. G., The Golden Bough, The Killing of the Divine Animal, Chapter LII.

18 Mythology of All Races,Vol. II p. 76.

19 Encyclopaedia of Religion & Ethics, Vol. VIII, p. 616, T & T Clarke, Edinburgh, 1914.

20 Ibid.

21 Mythology of All Races, Vol. 7, p. 370 (part 6.) Moses of Kalankata, History of Albaniap, 39–42.

22 Ibid., Vol. 7, p. 26.

23. Cumont, Franz, The Mysteries of Mithra, p. 179, Dover Publications Inc., NY, 1956.

24. Jung, C. G., Collected Works, Vol. 5, para. 669, Routledge & Kegan Paul, London.

2

THE RÔLE OF THE SKIN
IN THE OLD TESTAMENT

There are countless references in the Old Testament to the organ of the skin, both human and animal.

In the book of Exodus[1] it is said, "it came to pass when Moses came down from Mount Sinai with the two tablets of testimony in his hand, that Moses wist not, that the skin of his face shone while he talked with Him!" Then[2] "The children of Israel saw Moses, behold the skin of his face shone and they were afraid to come nigh him!" Later[3] it was necessary for Moses to veil his face.

It is apparent that the light which shone from Moses' face was great, since the phenomenon is described repeatedly, and it appears to have dazzled the eyes of the beholders. The verb 'to shine' with its past participle 'shone' in the English language is derived from the common Teutonic and Old English verb scinan, (scan, scinon, scinen). Each in turn is derived from the Old Testament root, skinan, and is undoubtedly connected with the roots of the word skin. Its meanings are to shed light, to give out light, and to illuminate or be radiant. It also has the meaning, of the day and the dawn. There is the added connotation, that is to be effulgent with splendour or beauty.

Thus the face of Moses was transfigured by his encounter with God; and in the language of primitive peoples from an earlier age, it would be said to radiate mana, the universal power of God. This also conjures up the very ancient idea that light was equivalent to both sight, and seeing.

The emotion engendered in Moses, by his meeting with God, was intensified to such an extent, that a physical affect became apparent in the shining of the face. The expression upon Moses' countenance was formed by

44

the indelible experience, whose effects were most certainly visible to others, since it was caused by a demonstrable change in personality. Jung[4] points out that when such events do occur "psychologically they betoken only a potential change, since they must be incorporated into consciousness, the accomplishment of which sometimes extends over long periods of time".

Moses' sister Miriam was likewise afflicted with a skin complaint, not exactly of the same nature as that of her brother.

The story of Miriam's punishment[5] following her sin reveals that she was smitten with leprosy and her skin became "as white as snow". Miriam herself a prophetess[6] was the elder sister of Moses, who sang at the Red Sea. Because her brother married an Ethiopian woman Miriam murmured against him. Her sin was two-fold, she was jealous of her brother's ability to prophesy, and because he married a foreigner. Jealousy always aims to pull down and destroy, and is a mortal sin. Miriam's name in Hebrew, means fat, thick and strong, so she probably represented a powerful maternal type of older sister for Moses.

When her leprosy appeared, this was followed at the dictate of God, by isolation from the camp for a period of seven days. Seven is the number which signifies transition. The leprous skin reflected the jealousy which possessed her and of which she was unconscious. It was thus the stigmata of her own malign nature directed against her younger brother. The 'lightness' of the skin denotes a potential illumination taking place in her soul. Thus the disease was a pointer to the inner darkness which required enlightenment. Her consciousness was in need of expansion regarding her own inner nature.

Moses was transfigured by the inner light of gnosis, psychologically a reflection of the light of the Self. Jung[7] says concerning such an encounter, "One should understand that the visualization of the Self is a 'window' into eternity".

In the book of Job, the skin again plays a rôle. In this book[8] one learns that Job was a man of Uz he was perfect, and upright and he feared God, eschewing evil. He lived harmoniously with his wife, children, servants and animals on his lands.

One day because of Satan's infamy God decided to beset Job with a multitude of disasters. The sorely tried Job lost all that he held dear, yet because of his innate nature, he bore all his calamities bravely, and did not speak against God. The final affliction brought to his servant by God was by the hand of his son Satan, and it was a skin disease.[9] Job was "smote with boils from the sole of his foot to the crown of his head". The onset of this dire disease caused his wife[10] to exhort her husband thus, "Dost thou still retain thy integrity? "Curse God and die".

This development, the onset of the dermatosis however was to be a landmark in the drama, as it marked the beginning of Job's confrontation with God. There are several references in the book of Job to the skin disorder but it is not possible to deduce its exact nature.

Job says of himself [11] "My flesh is clothed with worms and clods of earth, my skin is broken and becomes loathsome".

Later on[12] he exclaims "My bone cleaveth to my skin and to my flesh and I am escaped by the skin of my teeth". In his lamentations he is to cry out[13] "And though after my skin, worms destroy this body, yet in my flesh I shall see God". Finally[14] there is another pertinent remark "My bones are burned with heat".

One is able to conjecture from these remarks, and others that Job suffered from a widespread pustular, infective dermatosis characterised by heat or burning fever which led to gross emaciation with loss of flesh. Its initiation appears to have been fulminating as evidenced by the description of the explosive eruption of boils. The allusion to worms is referable to his impending death which was expected by Job, but of course there is a possibility that a maggot infestation did occur, as it does so often in hot desert or warm humid climates where chronic infection of whatever nature affects the skin. The life threatening, severe and generalised skin disease undoubtedly brought extreme physical suffering and abject mental anguish, as happens to all those dermatological invalids who are to be found, everywhere in the world, at every level of society.

In a human being the actual structure of the skin is subject to a constant turnover and renewal of its cells, as they grow from the innermost stratum germinativum, mature and reach the outer surface of the epidermis to form the hard stratum corneum or horny layer to be shed at a constant rate. This is quite unlike the skin of a reptile which is shed in totalis at approximately one year intervals. Thus the skin is a true organ of transformation, since it transforms itself from birth to death during every moment of its life in the greater life of the individual.

It has become apparent whilst exploring the rôle of the skin amongst primitive peoples, and in primitive thought that the skin is equated with the soul. Thus one is permitted to assume that the development of a skin disease points indubitably to a state of disorder, or a derangement in the relationship between ego consciousness (conscious psyche) and unconscious psyche. The psyche or the soul consists of both conscious and unconscious components.

In brief the soul becomes mislaid or has fallen into dereliction, abandoned or lost entirely, to the individual concerned, who thus is dissociated from his inner instinctual self. A state which at least is dangerous for the one who suffers it.

A skin disease such as is ascribed to Job is virtually a form of flaying in that the entire old skin is dying and must be cast off for renewal. The torture of flaying alive can only be accompanied by the most exquisite pain as is realized in the plebeian circumstance when a relatively small portion of skin is accidentally torn from the body. Job's anguish therefore was twofold, there was the physical pain and the psychological conflict occasioned by

God's injustice. The conflict became visible in the dermatosis and as the final affliction it represented the potential emergence of the conflict from the deepest layers of psyche, into consciousness. Job was confronted by the evidence in his own person of the need for a change of attitude, and a new awareness concerning the nature of his God.

In explanation concerning Job's conflict, Jung[15] has this to say "Job suffered under the powers of God and Satan, and became the unsuspecting plaything of two superhuman forces". Since Job[16] "is not conscious of this conflict in his own soul he never ceases to inveigh against the arguments of his friends who want to convince him of the evil in his own heart". Job is not conscious of the two great forces of good and evil but his whole life situation was destroyed by the dark side of God, who is called by us, the devil. As Jung[17] points out "this God dwells in the heart, in the unconscious, that is the source of our fear of the unspeakably terrible, and of the strength to withstand the terror".

The drama of Job portrays the torment of a soul punished by the bombardment of unconscious desires. Job had to realize that God's behaviour from a human view point was intolerable, and was that of a non-human being possessed of the dynamis of an elemental force. It was this force, total inexorable and unjust which confronted Job. His supreme task was to become conscious that God's behaviour as Jung[18] puts it, was that of "an unconscious being who cannot be judged morally".

The development of such a conflict and the extraordinarily difficult task of assimilation of its meaning for Job produced a prolonged period of suffering. The ensuing struggle was mirrored exactly in the process of the skin disease as it presented itself in various stages of decomposition, dissolution, putrefaction and lastly dessication. The skin became the visible expression of the transformation of energic process as the potentiality of a new consciousness replaced the former archaic attitude.

In these three biblical examples, it is apparent that it is the unconsciousness of a violent emotion, an inner desire or a torment of the soul in each of the individuals concerned. The skin condition reflects exactly, even precisely, the inner situation, the transfiguration of Moses, the dark evil of his sister and the torment of Job's moral conflict. The appearance of the skin change represents the outer visible manifestations of the inner problem whereby the flow of psychic libido is obstructed by the unconscious inner content.

REFERENCES

1 Old Testament, Exodus, Chapter 34, Verse 29.
2 Ibid., Verse 31.
3 Ibid., Verse 35.
4 Jung, C. G., Collected Works, Vol. X para 643.
5 Old Testament, Numbers, Chapter 12, V. 1–15.
6 Old Testament, Exodus, Chapter 15, V. 20.
7 Jung, C. G., Collected Works, Vol. 14 para 763.
8 Old Testament, Book of Job, Chapter 1, Verse l.
9 Old Testament, Book of Job, Chapter 2, Verse 7.
10 Ibid., Verse 9.
11 Ibid., Chapter 7, V. 5.
12 Ibid., Chapter l9, V. 20.
13 Ibid., Chapter19, V. 26.
14 Ibid., Chapter 30, V. 30.
15 Jung, C. G., Collected Works, Vol. 5. para 84.
16 Ibid. para 86.
17 Ibid. para 89.
18 Jung, C. G., Collected Works, Vol. II para 600.

3

THE RÔLE OF THE SKIN
IN FAIRY TALES

As has been observed the importance of the animal in the life of primitive man cannot be emphasised too cogently. The slow acceptance of Christian belief over the centuries and its increasing ubiquity has pushed the world of nature with her varied animal life to the periphery of mankind's collective conscious awareness.

The great changes wrought during the last two centuries in Western Europe and which included the migration of farm dwellers to the towns and cities together with the subsequent loss of the horse as a major means of transport has severed the age-old bond between man and beast. The loss is of the greatest magnitude for the future of man himself.

A mundane but salutary example, reported quite frequently is of the child who cannot relate to the fact of a packaged lamb cutlet upon the shelf of a supermarket, to the woolly sheep in the country fields. Since today very few people in the towns and cities ever see a dead animal in the streets, the fact of death particularly in the young is relegated to the outer limits of consciousness. Even the nature of human death is beyond comprehension in some instances. For example a medical doctor was called to a young woman of nineteen years who became hysterical when her grandmother died. Later she told the doctor that she did not know that people died. (One recalls the primitive myth of the cast skin.) The girl, an inner city dweller lived all her life in the soulless canyons of concrete, where no tree or flower bloomed. Hard as this is to believe, in the light of loss of contact with the instinctual life, it is understandable.

When an animal appears in a dream or a fantasy it usually represents an unconscious animal instinct which often may be dangerously primitive and threatening and yet on the obverse side of the coin it may signify a source of vital energy which has become lost to the conscious personality. Animals represent the dark unconscious aspects of psyche where man is archaic, primitive and, or barbarous. The instincts especially important are the group instinct, the urge to reproduce and the instinct of aggression.

The specific animal appearing in a dream is singularly important, it may be a wild and dangerous beast such as a lion, loose in the cellars of the dreamer's house. Or it may be a cunning fox, a charging rhinoceros or a cruising shark. All of these depict specific instinctual images, the meaning of which is unknown to the dreamer. So in fact when one sleeps one has the possibility to enter again the lost animal world, but because it is ignored, rejected or indeed is unknown, has become ominous and perhaps destructive for the dreamer. Often the animal may possess special qualities of great value indicating the sacred nature of the animal instinctuality long since deprived of conscious recognition. One calls to mind the healing dog and the divine serpent of the Greek god of doctors Asklepios.

For example a professional woman who worked very hard in a compulsive driven way, was possessed of a desire always to help others. She was very practical and gave of her best in a particularly unstinting indeed generous way. Her inferior function was intuition, and therefore she had difficulty in limiting herself. One night she dreamed that she was walking slowly with a heavy tread, head and shoulders bowed, and in her arms she was carrying an old dog who was dying of fatigue. This beautiful dream image says everything.

A woman had been forced into a difficult situation whereby she had become alienated from her inner world. She developed a pyrexia which seemed to have no known cause but which produced a constant subjective feeling of malaise. A few nights after the onset of the illness she dreamed she was lying in her own bed, upon a sumptuous fur blanket composed of beautiful cat skins. The next morning she was completely better.

The cat as symbol, par excellence, of feminine independence, was chosen by the unconscious to depict the compensation needed for the cure of her psychic estrangement. The fur blanket became a cloak composed of the qualities from which she had distanced herself.

In fairy stories, an important recurring theme is that of bewitchment of beings and who have been turned into animals. Such a theme occurs in Beauty and the Beast, where integration and humanization of the animal instincts is required. Sometimes very long periods of time pass before deep irrational emotions can be integrated into consciousness. This will be observed in some of the case material of modern individuals which is to be explored presently.

When such a curse occurs, the being concerned must go through the process of redemption before he or she is eventually changed back into a prince or princess. Von Franz[1] says:

"A human being in a neurotic state may be compared to a bewitched person, for people caught in a neurosis are apt to behave in a manner uncongenial and destructive towards themselves as well as others, they are forced onto too low a level of behaviour and act in an unconscious driven way. During the process of redemption, whereby the curse is overcome a common motif which is found quite frequently is where an individual has to wear an animal skin or an especial kind of skin has to be thrown over the being concerned. However to throw a skin over someone is also another way of applying a curse. Thus the individual can be both redeemed and cursed by a skin thrown over him or her."

She continues:[2]

"Practically this means that a complex of psyche which has human means of expression is so depotentiated that it has only animal means of expression. In such a case the individual with such a complex is robbed of human expression a condition which is associated with compulsive driveness."

A woman with a severe mother complex suffered dreadfully all her life from the inability to express herself. In middle life as old age faced her, she dreamed she was confronted by a polar bear, standing upright on his hind legs. Strangely she said she did not feel fear. In fact, in the dream she behaved exactly as she would have done in reality, she remained mute. Such was the brutalizing effect of the violent emotions engendered in her psyche. In her case that which was potentially human, a cry, a shout or a step backwards did not occur. Such a human instinct denoting a reaction of terror before the unknown was obliterated. She was, so to speak turned to stone overcome by the violent opposing emotions engendered in psyche. One would be permitted to say a "bewitchment" occurred by an act of vengeance on the part of a witch resulting in a descent into the wild animal.

Many years were to pass before a dream occurred in which she bought herself a protective coat made of fur skins which she wore with pride because it was her own.

REFERENCES

1 Von Franz, The Psychological Meaning of Redemption Motifs in Fairy Tales, p. 8, Inner City Books, Toronto, Canada.
2 Ibid., p. 42.

PART II

In the following exposition of the various and several skin diseases and disorders encountered in the general practice of dermatology a brief explanation of the morbid condition is appended. However this treatise is not a textbook of dermatology.

It is a means to investigate and render conscious, the unconscious psychic background of a number of dermatological victims who presented themselves in order to seek health.

The case material provides a number of examples, to illustrate each of the specific and common somatic conditions described. Certain similarities will undoubtedly be observed between some of the individual case histories. However it would be unwise to conclude that a certain archetypal presence, or the activation of a common complex indubitably leads to the appearance of the same skin condition in different human beings. The great danger inherent in the use of case material is to seek a common cause or a collective solution to a specific problem, as indeed is the case in general medicine. It must be stressed that in each of the described life histories, an individual solution was sought for the problem in each case, no matter what the skin disease.

In order to ensure anonymity only the age, sex, and where relevant the occupation of the individual has been supplied.

4

ECZEMA

This disorder of the skin accounts for a large proportion of all skin disease. It is induced by a wide range of factors, both internal and external. When the cause is thought to be external to the body, due to infections, irritants and allergic contacts, the eczema is said to be exogenous in character. If the eczema is induced internally it is described as endogenous, and a result of constitutional factors.

Eczema is a distinctive pattern of inflammatory response. Its histopathological features, reflect a dynamic sequence of changes which results in an inflammation of the epidermis, and the underlying structures. Thus when one speaks of eczema, it is of an inflammatory process which accounts for the increased warmth and swelling, discomfort, and not the least, irritation. The essential lesion. of whatever type is the primordial vesicle, which is a tiny blister, and is crucial to the diagnosis. It is situated in the mid-epidermal region. The dynamis of eczema consists of a series of events, described as stages. However they merge and inter-merge so rapidly that it is impossible to observe them clinically. All that is visible is a damaged red, scaly or oozing skin. The first stage of papulation eases quickly into the stage of vesiculation. As the vesicles erupt, exudation intercedes, followed by crusting of the sero-exudate, and scaling. The process is eternally recurring until and when healing intervenes. The primordial vesicle is an infinitessimally tiny volcano in the process of erupting through the skin. When there is thousands-fold multiplication the end result is a patch of eczema. The word itself, has been in use in the English language since the mid-eighteenth century, but it is derived from the Greek word which means 'to boil'. The word is excellent in its exactitude.

If a psychological assessment can be undertaken in all presenting cases of the disorder, of either classification, it becomes clear that, in by far and away, the majority of all patients, the psychic background is of singular pertinence. Particularly is this so, when reviewed against the specific type of eczema which develops, and its siting on the body. The time factor, together with the primordial vesicle is likewise always crucial, but its establishment usually requires patience and persistence on the part of the physician, and frankness and willingness to participate on the side of the sufferer.

Eczema commonly affects the hands. Nowhere is this more apparent than in the modern industrial world. The disadvantages hinge upon loss of livelihood, but the advantages of compensation often far outweigh the former. The frequency of complete recovery against all apparent odds, after the settlement of legal strife, is an aspect not to be ignored and requires circumspection. In the industrial realm the psychic background of the workman is unlikely to be considered, the diagnosis of hand eczema is rationalized to a specific cause of contact or allergen at work. The fact that the workman is a human individual with family life outside his job, and an inner psychic life of instincts and emotions is not to be entertained. Yet, this unconscious world is as vital to him as that of external reality. When it is unconscious to him, and unconscious really does mean not conscious, the dangers inherent are infinitely greater. The questions which are not asked are: Why this disease? Why the hands? and Why this time?

An engineer workman develops an irritant eczema of the hands. This is believed to be due entirely to a new cutting oil or coolant fluid used on the machines, which has been recently introduced at work. He does not correlate the skin condition with the fact that he is about to divorce his wife, or perhaps he has just discovered that his mistress is unfaithful to him, or he has learned that his son is a hopeless drug addict, or that his mother has died. If he is aware at all of his associated psychic distress he usually does not relate it spontaneously to his working life and the concomitant hand eczema. The condition becomes either prolonged or chronic, until such time as a psychic transformation occurs and the inner emotion is either realized or more often it again slips away deeper into unconsciousness, to appear perhaps sometime in future years, in another form. Consciousness of inner emotional life, however it seems, is an obligation required by the Self.

Again perhaps a man has worked for the rubber industry for forty years, in the company of thousands of men. One morning he awakens with eczema of the hands. Skin patch tests prove that he has an undoubted allergy to the chemicals of rubber. Investigations as to the time factor reveal that the day on which the skin "broke down weeping" was the day which followed the sad news that his much loved wife of many years had an intractable disease and would die within weeks. A housewife develops an irritant hand eczema possibly due to the washing up detergents or cleaning materials. If enquiry is made it is discovered that there is a coincidental unconscious dread, springing from the negative emotional reaction associated with the added burden of the advent of a new baby, or the unwanted intrusion of a helpless aged relative, into the home. A schoolboy develops an allergy to leather lining of his school shoes, which produces a severe eczema of the soles of the feet, (the sole of the foot is that part in closest contact with the reality world). To be precise he has developed a hypersensitivity reaction to the metal chromium, which is used to cure leather. Only later is it realized that the sudden allergy coincided with his promotion to a higher class at school, where he found himself at odds with a tyrannical school master. He had been put 'upon his metal'.

A woman of middle years suffers a reaction to an expensive perfume within a day or so of using it for the first time. Then she recalls that it was the gift of a lover who jilted her in shocking circumstances, six months previously. He had given her the perfume as a parting gift. Her skin rejected it, because she had 'forgotten' the psychic rejection of the man himself.

Another woman who had held a prestigious job in the world of fashion fell upon hard times, and was reduced to being a cashier in a down town bar where the hours were long, and the customers jaded. She developed a hand eczema, and it was proved that she had an allergy to nickel the metal in the money which she 'handled' constantly, and which she regarded as dirty. Her hands rejected the job, because she was unaware of the force of her psychic resistance to her new earning capacity. All of these physical conditions were classified as exogenous eczema having apparently an external cause, but the coincidental psychic factors were of paramount importance.

A small girl of five years developed an eczema of the palm of the right hand. It was regarded as constitutional, without a visible cause. It began the day after she had gone to school for the first time. She had had to relinquish the protective hand of her mother, which she had been holding tightly. Such a child of tender years was not able to express one syllable denoting distress or fear, and so she remained mute, before the approach of the unknown. Some time later it became evident that on that day it was the mother herself who had repressed her fears and had unconsciously transmitted them to the child with whom she had identified.

In men, the hands represent primarily the ability to work and to a lesser extent to support, whereas with women, whose principle of Eros is one of feminine relatedness, the hands signify the capacity to grasp and to hold. In all the cases described, ego consciousness was faced with an apparently insuperable obstacle, 'the hands were tied', and psychically an obstruction to the flow of libido had developed. It is very important to consider the ubiquitous problem of all eczemas from the psychic view point as well as the physical.

The eczematous process initiated by the presence of the primordial vesicle is an identical reflection in miniature of that of a volcanic explosive catastrophe. In terms of reference for the human dermatological invalid the damage is equivalent. The planetary event releases the build up of tension from the combustible gaseous materials in the subterranean realm. It is therefore not unreasonable to relate the human process to an increase of inner psychic tension, such as occurs when an archetype is constellated in the unconscious.

Jung defines an archetype as a nuclear dynamism of the psyche, resembling a mass of dynamic energy. The skin of the individual, as does the earth's crust, acts as a safety valve, appearing to permit the release of tension, through the dynamis of the eczematous process, or explosion.

Each of the cases of hand eczema mentioned briefly above, exhibit the development of a skin disorder, and the presence of an unconscious psychic factor causally unrelated, but related in time. As such they are synchronistic events. Jung[1] in his article on synchronicity says that "causality is the way we explain the link between two successive events, but synchronicity designates the parallelism of time and meaning between psychic and psychophysical events, which scientific knowledge so far has been unable to reduce to a common principle".

He continues[2] "no reciprocal causal connection can be shown to obtain between parallel events, which is just what gives them their chance character". Such events cannot be predicted or foreseen since they are not regular. In Jung's view synchronistic events were manifestations of a causal orderedness, which occurs to a certain extent in nature. Von Franz[3] describes these as "certain orders which physical and psychic nature keep, thus producing by those constant events, a constant order".

Synchronistic events are unique acts of creation in time. Perhaps a remarkable event which is to be described may illustrate this.

THE GIRL WITH THE MUMMIFIED HANDS.

One afternoon at about two o'clock a young woman of twenty-two years, came by way of her physician, with a chronic eczema of the hands. She was exceedingly pleasant, intelligent, and anxious to know if anything could help her. She had undoubtedly a hand condition but it was part of an eczematous process affecting her whole body which is classed as Atopic dermatitis and is often thought to be constitutional. She had been the victim of this condition since two days after her birth. She had sought advice, because she was a check-out girl at a supermarket, and was ashamed of her hands, which were dry, wrinkled and scaly. In my view they resembled the hands of a mummified corpse.

Her anamnesis was not remarkable and the family situation seemed to be without problems. She was the only daughter, and had an exceedingly close attachment to her mother whom she loved dearly. Since she was of the opinion that little could be done, she was therefore not inclined to dawdle, when I told her that I could offer nothing new in the way of treatment, which would be of lasting benefit for her condition. For some minutes she asked questions about the cause of her lifelong condition. She had been told that it was inherited. As she prepared to leave I had an intuition that I should explain to her the psychic background of the disorder, as I had experienced it over the years, in my practice. We dwelt for a little while on the fact of her lack of friends, and the close relationship with her mother. It was explained very briefly that as much as she loved her mother, such a close bond could be damaging, since it is always to a lesser or greater extent, restricting for the individuals concerned, both for the mother and the daughter, but particularly for the latter. She departed, and it seemed to me that I had not explained the mother archetype as clearly as I might have done. I believed that she had not exactly understood my homily. However some weeks later she returned, her condition was in the main unchanged, except for a certain liveliness of disposition which I had not perceived on the former occasion.

She opened the conversation with the remark that although her skin was much about the same, she knew that she was going to get completely well. The reason was that something wonderful had happened, and that is why she knew she had been cured.

After leaving me, she had gone straight home, and had arrived there, about a quarter to five o'clock. She removed her coat, and went into the kitchen to boil some water for her tea. Whilst waiting for the kettle to boil, standing there in the kitchen, she was suddenly overcome with a desperate fatigue. It was so great that she could no longer stand, and she had to sit down in a chair, at the kitchen table. She looked at the clock as she did so, and it was five minutes to five o'clock. She fell asleep and had a most extraordinary and vivid dream, which woke her up. When she looked at the clock it was one minute to five o'clock so the deep sleep, the dream, and the awakening had all taken place in a period of four minutes. In the dream she was in a place underground, where there were many passages. She realized that she had never been in such a place before, but she knew what the place was, for whilst she was actually in the place, she also had a vision of it in her mind's eye. When she got up she felt quite refreshed and decided to draw the dream which she brought to me eventually. This in itself was remarkable as the question of dreams had not been discussed between us. The drawing of the dream was small but very intricate. It had been executed on a small piece of rough, lined, off-white paper. To my astonishment it was an elaborate and circular labyrinth, and at the centre of it was a tiny figure of a naked woman in a recumbent posture. That was the dream. As we studied the drawing together I asked her if she had any idea what it was, she said that it was a labyrinth, the woman in the drawing was not she, herself, but related to her in some way, and that woman, which she had drawn, lived there, in the labyrinth. I gave her back the picture, because it was a testament of truth from the unconscious. As I looked at her vibrant face, she said 'I am cured, it is a miracle'. Indeed I agreed with my full consciousness. At that moment we both knew that the neurosis was resolving, and her skin would recover. I never saw her again.

The labyrinth is essentially an intercrossing of paths, many of which are cul-de-sacs and it is thus a question of finding the route which leads to the centre. This was the problem for Theseus who escaped the Minotaur dwelling in the great labyrinth at Knossos. Often the labyrinth is engraved on the floors, walls and tombs of pre-history. At Cumae the sanctuary of the Sibylle had a labyrinth engraved on the door. It is found all over the world from Europe to China. The passage from the entrance to the centre represents an initiation, a voyage of discovery, and was forbidden to all but those who were authorized to enter. The labyrinth is associated with the mandala which also has the aspect of the labyrinth, both have the hidden centre. In nature the dance of the bees, and certain dances of birds particularly storks as found in China, reconstruct the pattern of the labyrinth. In them, is a natural ordered plan of nature itself, and is an archetypal image. The labyrinth is also a system of defence, it announced the presence of something unknown, something secret, hithertofore unrecognised and therefore sacred. This is why access was permitted only to the initiated. The secret lay in the centre which was reserved for the initiant, who was to be privy to the revelation of the mystery.

The labyrinth in the girl's drawing was in the form of a circle and was a mandala.[4] This is a Sanskrit word meaning circle, and magic circle. The most important forms are concentrically arranged figures or round or square patterns with a centre. Jung[5] says that the mandala as a symbol of unity occurs as a compensation of the contradictions and conflicts of the conscious situation. As the ultimate oneness of all archetypes it is a secret oneness, the central figure in the drawing symbolized both the centre of the labyrinth, and the centre of the mandala. This represents therefore both the oneness and the totality. Jung[6] says "unity and totality stand at the highest point on the scale of objective values because their symbols can no longer be distinguished from the imago Dei". He goes on to say[7] that "individual mandalas are symbols of order occurring in those who suffer psychic disorientation, or (are in need) of reorientation".

Thus this young woman slept and dreamed, and for a moment of wholeness glimpsed eternity, and the ineffable and infinite mystery of the Self. The skin disease, lifelong, was the physical manifestation of the disordered relationship between her mother and herself. Behind the maternal archetype, but eternally present was the archetype of order and wholeness, that of the Self. The archetypal image in the dream was the transformation, and the girl understood. She perceived unconsciously the harmony and the equilibrium lacking in her outer life.

The afternoon was a synchronistic event. It was the time for her to seek healing, it was also the time for her to be sought by the Self. The dried and mummified-corpse hands symbolised the death hold of the mother arche-type in her life. But were to lead her to the reactivation and by the grace of God, eventual re-integration of her own feminine wholeness.

ATOPIC DERMATITIS*

In the previous case, it was found the young woman had suffered from this disorder all her life. It is usually described as Atopic dermatitis instead of eczema because true eczematous changes are not always present. Atopy is believed to be a genetically determined disorder in which there is an increased liability to form reagin (IgE) antibodies, and an increased susceptibility to certain diseases especially asthma, hay fever, and Atopic dermatitis. To describe the latter condition as "allergic eczema is quite misleading, constitutional eczema imprecise, and disseminated neuro-dermatitis emphasises only one aspect of its aetiology".[8]

The fundamental defects remain unknown. The sufferers have an inherently irritable skin, they do not sit well in their skins. The condition usually starts early in life between two and six months, the age of two days as described in the case history above is exceptional, but does occur. It is a chronic fluctuating disease and itching is the cardinal symptom. It is always accompanied by considerable distress on the part of the affected child, it was described in the past as a 'milestone' disorder. It had been observed by medical attendants that the child usually recovered, or went into a prolonged remission, when he went to school, or later to senior school, college, university, into an occupation or joined the armed services. In other words when a major displacement from home took place. On the other hand it was also noted that after an apparent recovery or remission, exacerbations occurred when any new ventures were undertaken. These Included engagement, marriage, the advent of a child or divorce.

The disease may start at any time of life even after fifty years, but usually tends to disappear with age. The skin becomes leathery dry and excoriated because of constant traumata through scratching. It has a characteristic picture and in childhood presents a disturbing image. The baby or the young child is unhappy, it cries constantly, scratches perpetually and is a miserable and dejected little creature. In short, a child perhaps difficult to love. Indubitably this is a factor which may affect adversely, the mother's attitude towards it. A suggestion which often is denied. Another feature commonly observed in early childhood is an uncontrolled 'possessed' curiosity which sometimes amounts to manic proportions. It is often accompanied by a distinct will to destructiveness behind a show of timidity. There is another aspect which may not easily be ignored, it is a tendency on the part of the child to cling to its mother, refusing to leave her. Yet after a display of affection, the mother may be dealt a savage blow to her person by the offspring, who promptly falls, into a screaming rage. Such ambivalence is pronounced and observed not infrequently.

Atopic dermatitis is a common disorder, and constitutes a great problem in dermatology. However it is an undisputed fact that as soon as atopic children are admitted to hospital or clinics for care, their skins clear at once and revert to a relative normality, in a matter of days. On discharge to their homes after recovery, there is almost always a reversal to the former state. This fact has always seemed to me to be of the utmost significance.

It was this observation which led me eventually to pay strict attention to the psychology of the parents, in particular that of the mother of these children. It became evident that there was an unconscious maternal rejection factor. This ties in with the observed pattern and progression of the disease process, and fits in with the milestone theory of the early years. It seems that the child is unsure of the mother, because the mother is ambivalent towards the child. In later years, a pattern develops in which the individual himself incorporates the pattern of maternal rejection, and the negative effects of the maternal archetype dominate all aspects of life. The individual both accepts and rejects himself. He is always hesitant concerning the future, and tends to glance backwards to the past. Unconsciously he seeks approbation, support and encouragement from the 'the mother'. This accounts for the hesitancy and exacerbations in mature years following remission, when an unexpected transitional stage presents itself.

(1) THE CLOWN BOY

This child came when he was five years old. His mother explained that he had developed atopic eczema at the age of two weeks. He was severely afflicted and unusually withdrawn and silent in manner. Later at all times, he appeared to me to be very miserable. In an adult such a condition would be described as a severe depression. His skin was eczematous and infected because of the constant scratching and tearing by the fingers. There was also a perioral eczema, a thick rim of inflammatory reaction all round the mouth, which was inflamed, red in colour, fissured and bleeding. It had the appearance of the vividly painted lips and greatly accentuated mouths of circus performers. He looked like a sad little clown. This reaction had resulted from the habit of constantly licking his lips, which gave him both a fearful and furtive demeanour.

His mother's manner towards him was distant, she did not address him, look at him or acknowledge him, it was as if he did not exist. He was however well nourished, suitably clothed and cared for physically. There is no gainsaying his appearance was singularly unprepossing, and I myself felt disinclined to expend more than a modicum of energy upon him. Treatment for the condition was ordered and he returned a few weeks later without improvement. This is not an infrequent occurrence in skin clinics.

On the occasion of his second visit I decided to speak to the mother and dismissed the child to the care of an attendant, requesting as I did so, a glass of milk and a biscuit for him. At once the mother sprang to her feet and adamantly declared that he was not to be given a biscuit. I was astonished at her sudden ferocity. When enquiry was made as to the reason for the denial, she said that his teeth must be preserved. It came to light that the boy had never received anything of a sweet nature, neither bonbon, chocolate or pudding in his entire life. It was at that moment that I realized that the mother was possessed of a powerful animus which was a force to be reckoned with indeed. The opinions of the animus, the masculine unconscious psyche of a woman, are usually just wide of the mark. In this case admirable though it was to preserve the child's dentition, circumspection was required, and a degree of licence permitted. The child received his first chocolate biscuit that day, both to his surprise and pleasure.

The only hope for any degree of improvement in his condition rested in a change of attitude on the mother's part. Fortunately in our subsequent conversation together, she did admit frankly that the child had not been wanted, and was for her an unwelcome incubus. She and her husband had been married for several years before the baby was conceived. The husband was a well known sportsman and the couple lived an extrovert social life, travelling constantly, to various countries. The woman said that her husband had a weakness for the opposite sex and when she was not with him she was always afraid that he might be unfaithful, and find someone to replace her. Therefore whenever possible she always made it her business to accompany him. Furthermore she added that she had always known that her husband had no feeling for family life. The child's imminence disrupted this life and the husband began to travel alone, the woman remaining at home. At once she began to resent the child in utero. Two weeks after the birth, the eczema started, and soon the entire body was affected. During the subsequent five years, fluctuations occurred but the skin had never cleared.

The perioral reaction had begun a few weeks earlier when he had gone to school. The mother insisted that the father never took any interest In the child. It seemed at the same time that this remark possibly emanated from the animus. This assumption on my part, however, was later to be corroborated when I discovered that the boy and his father had an excellent rapport albeit the father was often absent from home.

It soon became apparent that the child had severe nightmares, these were discussed and he agreed to draw pictures of the things which frightened him at night. His mother added the information that the scratching was always worse in the night when he was asleep. When he returned after this discussion he and his mother entered the room in reasonably good spirits, and it was clear, that the mother for once, was amused. She said immediately, "he has brought a picture which he has drawn for you, it is a witch and he

63

said it is me!" The drawing consisted of a cooking pot and hovering over it was a witch in a tall cap, with a long nose. In her right hand was a stick. She was cooking the dinner, and stirring the pot with the stick. In the pot was not the dinner but a little boy. The child solemnly explained in his mother's presence that the witch was his mother, and he was the little boy. This was the dream which had frightened him the most. In the astounded silence which ensued I looked at the mother's smiling face, and the serious face of the boy. The immense and prophetic statement was made in total incomprehension of its significance by both the boy and the mother.

Then I hugged the boy spontaneously, there was nothing else to be done. From that moment, our relationship got off to a flying start. In the following weeks he produced shoals of drawings, usually of dreams or anything which caught his interest. The therapy consisted merely of looking at his drawings, with one or two remarks. Nothing was ever explained to him. The mother endured these sessions, and seemed to consider them a waste of time or possibly her animus did. But she did bring him regularly and she did see that he brought the drawing book, each visit.

After about three years the child had recovered. He was by then eight years old, and had in fact outgrown his fears; indeed he had outgrown his mother.

This boy had the misfortune to be born to a woman who rejected him as soon as she learned she was pregnant, and she refused to accept him after birth. However the strong animus insisted that he was brought up rigorously and cared for suitably. She protected his teeth fiercely and repaired the ravaged skin. This is a perfect picture of a maternalism dominated by animus opinions. However it was a mechanical care, which was provided, without warmth, real thought, affection or any visible sign of relationship. She had an extraordinarily distant attitude, and one received the impression that she lived in a cocoon. At the time the extent of her animus possession was not realised, this came much later. This child was born into and brought up in an atmosphere of unconscious maternal rejection and hostility. He was the source of constant irritation for his mother, because he had intruded into her life and provided a threat to her stability. She was at base desperately afraid that her husband might prefer another woman, a fear not without foundation in view of her nature. The boy had therefore no standpoint in reality, for he was without any knowledge of what possible crime he had committed to deserve such a reception from life. He was trapped without escape, this accounted for the curiously fearful and furtive attitude. At night the unconscious provided images of his mother in the rôle of a lamia, and his days were filled with dread and an understandable mortal fear of life, which he was not able to formulate to anyone.

The positive feminine support which he received in therapy, his own drawing regarded without interpretation was all that was necessary to give him a reality standpoint. Since he had a firm relationship with his father he was able to discriminate and regard his mother objectively, and to accept her. When he left therapy it was clear that he would progress to normal masculine independence. His last visit produced a drawing of a bird's nest, in which a tiny fledgling had just hatched from an egg, its large mouth was opened wide. He had been born.

This recalled to me, the initial symptom which had long since disappeared. The perioral eczema had been exacerbated by the continual lip sucking. The mouth symbolizes the food intake and word output. The child had received no comforting sweetness, the warm milk of human kindness had been denied him by his mother. Similarly he could not express himself because of fear. The unconscious represented this by accentuating vividly the mouth and lips in the eczematous reaction, enclosing the area. The clown's lips indicated the necessity to formulate in words the underlying emotional distress. The drawings did this for him. Perhaps in spite of my profound doubts I hoped some impression had also been made upon the mother's animus, as the boy gradually overcame the fears which it had engendered.

The child as an image represented exactly the constant hostility, irritation, fear, and entrapment of his mother's unconscious personality. Had she had but the wit, she would have observed herself in that miserable helpless man-child.

Many years later I was to be involved in a series of epidemics of psychic possession among industrial workers.[9] In each of several epidemics, it was discovered that there was always a central dominant personality who instigated, and propagated the trouble. In one of the smaller (and unpublished) epidemics, the central figure was a woman. She had started with a skin rash on her hands, and had blamed the factory product, which was a cloth, as the cause. She sat at a central table in the factory and within weeks many of the workers at surrounding tables all developed eczema of the hands. Everyone was tested and found to be negative but the central figure of the epidemic did not appear for tests. After diligent searching she was found and tested. It was discovered that she alone of all the victims had a true hand eczema, due to the metal nickel, not the cloth she handled at work. Furthermore she had known that she had a true nickel eczema for several years, before she had undertaken work at the factory, and which she had concealed from her employers. When I eventually met her, I was surprised to discover that I already knew her, she was the mother of the clown boy. She had apparently remarried, and had another name, but I knew her face, at once.

The unconscious gave to her son the true picture of her personality, many years earlier. Without doubt she was a deeply unconscious woman.

(2) THE GIRL WITH THE
BLACK SNAKE SKIN BOOTS.

An ophthalmologist colleague requested that I examine a young girl of eleven years, suffering from a serious eye infection, as well as a generalised atopic dermatitis. She had a true atopic diathesis, having suffered from both eczema and asthma, since her birth. The two conditions usually alternated, but at the time of the eye infection, they were both present. The asthma was grave enough to warrant high dosage of steroid drugs, which did not contain the skin disorder.

The inflammation of the left eye had begun suddenly just after the mother of the child had returned from hospital with a newly born baby girl. The little patient confessed that her parents were delighted with the new baby because she had a 'perfect skin'. She said that she loved the baby very much, and added that she 'desperately' wanted to be a nurse. She was in hospital at the time. The following year, the mother brought the girl for dermatological advice. This was the only time I saw the mother. Psychotherapy was suggested as the best solution, and the mother agreed.

However the parents it seemed were gregarious and constantly moving house, so the suggestion fell by the wayside.

Eventually an able child-therapist took over her case, and for a time apparently she made some progress. I did not see her for some years.

When the girl was sixteen years old she returned again through the agency of her general physician because of the parlous state of the skin. It was then I discovered the sad neglect of the girl whose psychotherapy had been discontinued years before. The parents had a lucrative business which entailed long periods of absence from home. The young girl had been left solely with the responsibility of bringing up the younger sister, as well as her own welfare. After this visit she came regularly to see me for two years. During our conversations together it became evident that she wished me to believe that she held her parents in high esteem, she extolled their praiseworthy virtues stressing their generosity in paying for her treatment, their kindness and love for their children, particularly it seemed the baby sister. Since I had only met the mother once, the girl was either accompanied by a maid or came alone, and I had not encountered the father therefore I had no knowledge of them. It was clearly a fact that they played a central rôle in her life. I asked about dreams, but she did not have any, and in the two years she attended she was never able to recall a single dream.

After six months during which little progress was made I received a letter from her. In it was an outpouring of emotion, such as I have rarely witnessed in a communication from a patient. She declared that her parents were not what they seemed. They quarrelled constantly, and regularly fought with each other. On occasion they physically attacked each other, injuring and wounding themselves. Moreover they had done so, ever since she could remember. Although she expressed a fondness for her mother, she asserted that she hated her father. She wrote that "as a child I lay in bed at night, listening to them and quaking with terror". When this admission had been made things improved, possibly because I accepted the letter and its contained information without comment, and by so doing 'accepted' her. From that time we were able to discuss freely the apparently appalling state of affairs at home. She stressed that outward appearances belied the inner situation of the family.

By the time she reached the age of eighteen, she was much improved. The skin had resolved in a remarkable fashion, and the asthma was easily controlled. She enrolled as a nurse, and underwent a training course. She left home to live in a nursing students' hostel and at once a profound transformation occurred. Her respiratory infections abated, her spirits lifted and she began to enjoy the work and her colleagues' friendship.

It was some three years later when I saw her again, and found her vastly changed. She told me that she was about to marry an Indian doctor whom she had met recently. They were to live abroad after the marriage, and she was looking forward to it very much. Her parents apparently were delighted at the prospect, and her father liked the man (this should have been a warning). An unusual feature of the meeting which proved to be the last time I was to see her, was the way in which she was dressed. Her clothes from head to toe were of black leather, and her footwear consisted of black snake skin boots. The impact of her presence was electrifying and had a profoundly disturbing effect upon me. A feeling of foreboding overtook me, which I could not shake off.

She departed after receiving a further appointment to return before her marriage. She never kept it, for she fell and fractured a foot, and I did not see her again. Two years later I enquired of her progress from a colleague who had treated her asthma, but he had no information. Shortly afterwards the mother of the girl, having heard of my enquiry telephoned me to say that a year previously, that is a year after I had seen her, she had committed suicide. In the preceding year she had become addicted to barbiturates, and had taken an over-dose. The doctor did not marry her, and she had gone to live with an engineering student from the sub-continent as his fiancée.

The mother expressed no regret, at her daughter's death but praised the daughter's lover, and intimated how dreadful the whole affair had been for him. She spoke as if the girl was a stranger to her, as indeed she was. In the ten year period during which I saw the girl intermittently I only met the mother once, and the father not at all. This reveals a degree of unrelatedness and neglect of the girl herself as their child, and as a human being. No interest, nor even enquiry was forthcoming but the fees were paid regularly. If as the girl contended the home conditions were of such a nature, the inhuman quarrelling and abuse of the parents indicated a gross unconsciousness, and maladaptation of these adults. A child born into such a psychic atmosphere of violence, mistrust, and hatred could hardly be expected to thrive. In fact it was a small miracle that she lived so long, with her severe disability.

In retrospect it was significant that she developed a severe infection of the left eye at the age of eleven years, when her baby sister was born. Plotinus said that the eye would not be able to see the sun, if in a manner, it was not itself a sun. Seeing then represents illumination and understanding. Jung[10] says "the eye like the sun is a symbol as well as an allegory of consciousness". The Blind Stone[11] in Malekula meant that the eyes should be closed to the outer world so that the mind became conscious of inner events. The left eye as the moon represents moon consciousness or feminine consciousness. The eye condition and the exacerbation of the skin condition, together with the asthma, and the advent of the new sister all at the same time was a synchronistic event. The girl had not 'seen' and therefore was not aware of the meaning of the mother's joyful acceptance of the new child with 'the perfect skin'. The sick left eye which had closed, to outer reality was required to perceive an inner vision, a conscious realization of her own reality in the situation of the family with its lack of warm relatedness towards her. It was an opportunity to see that her skin condition (and also the asthma) emanated from her mother's unconscious rejection of herself as a person. This unconscious knowledge undoubtedly resulted in the 'desperate' need to become a nurse. The girl was in desperate need of being nursed herself.

The extraordinary change which occurred when she met the Indian lover was reflected in the donning of the dark clothes, with the black serpentine skin boots. The foreboding which I experienced was justified, she had fallen into the darkness of the unconscious shadow. In all probability in meeting the Indian student in the outer world, she met her unconscious animus, who proved to be both negative and destructive. On the occasion of her last visit she had lost her cheerfulness and appeared cold and distant, and somehow proud. Her standpoint in life had become detached from reality. She had lost her warmth and relatedness, a fact corroborated symbolically by the black snake skin boots. Bearing in mind at that time marriage was in the offing with the Indian doctor, it seems as if her outward meeting with him had initiated the descent into the dark mother.

She was a simple unsophisticated young invalid woman who through her own diligence had achieved a standpoint albeit precarious, in reality. A constellation of events, success in her studies, the flattering attentions of a worldly man had produced hubris. The injury to the foot indicates a loss of balance. Inflation is accompanied by an increase in unconsciousness, always a serious hazard, but for this young woman, a great danger.

Without precise details of her exact situation a tentative assumption is that she found herself once again, in the same plight which she had experienced under her parents' roof. Overpowered by her cold and unrelated shadow side, the realm of the interiorized parents, the frail ego consciousness perished, and with it sadly, her life.

(3) THE PUER AETERNUS

One of the hazards of atopic dermatitis is an eye affliction. Several varieties do occur, but most commonly and particularly in the young are those due to infection, self induced by scratching. Rubbing the irritable eyes can lead to coning of the cornea and also to cataract.

A man in his early forties, a printer by trade, had suffered from atopic dermatitis since the age of six months. His skin was severely affected, and the entire body was excoriated so that he appeared to be the victim of flagellation. About a year before he presented he had suffered a detachment of the retina of the left eye, with subsequent loss of sight. He was unmarried, and lived with his mother, his father having died when he was an adolescent. He explained that he had never married, because he had been unable to find the right wife. In any event he had to stay at home to care for his mother, who incidentally was both fit and well. He was an only child.

He looked younger than his age, was very pleasant, and at all times exhibited a benign equanimity. This belied the appearance of the skin, which in its fiery redness resembled a blazing inferno. The fact of the sudden loss of sight a year earlier, was taken seriously and enquiry made as to the circumstances of the events at the time. He was not able to offer anything in the way of preceding difficulties or problems prior to the event. The only thing of importance that he could recall was that at the time the detachment occurred, his skin had deteriorated profoundly, and it had remained in the same parlous state since.

The eye is circular and is a mandala signifying wholeness. As the organ of physical perception it is almost universally the symbol of intellectual perception. In the Bhagavad Gita the two eyes are identified with the sun and moon. Traditionally the right eye is the sun and corresponds to, day, activity and the future, the left eye is the moon and represents night, darkness, passivity, and the past. The Shamans always and still do in some areas, put coverings over their eyes. This was to symbolize a blindness to the outer world, and their concentration on their inner visions. Wotan the raging god, sacrificed an eye to Mimir in exchange for the gift of wisdom.

This man's condition warranted hospitalization, with care and therapy he began to improve. It became clear that the mother-son relationship was of the utmost importance and indeed urgency. He admitted that he himself had a weak character, and his mother dominated him. He said that he was really afraid of her anger, and her cold withdrawals. In short he found her both selfish and cruel, without a semblance of consideration for him. When it was asked why he did not leave her, he said he could not bear the guilt should she become ill or die. It was explained to him that his outer calmness was a façade, and the skin revealed a furious inner rage, which had been repressed for decades. The symbol of the volcano was presented, and struck a cord in his psyche, for he at once understood.

His mother never visited him whilst he was in hospital, but he was condemned to telephone her every evening. It was noticed that the evening temperature as well as his pulse rate and blood pressure levels were elevated after these telephonic communications. Yet in spite of repeated warnings he was unable to resist the compulsion. When the skin had improved sufficiently, he was referred to a psychotherapist, with his full and enthusiastic consent.

Shortly after his return home, cardiac symptoms intervened, and during the subsequent investigations, inexplicably, he died.

Puer Aeternus, means "eternal youth" and is the name of a god of antiquity. Ovid speaks of the child-god in the Eleusinian mysteries who is called Iacchus praising him in his rôle in the mysteries and addressing him as 'puer aeternus'[12]. The term is used to describe "a certain type of young man who has an outstanding mother complex[13]. The man who is identified with this archetype remains too long in the psychology of youthful adolescence, as he ages physically. This is combined with a too great dependence upon the mother. There is usually a severe ambivalence in the mother-son relationship.

The man admitted the difficulties with his mother, he also asserted that he could not find a woman to suit him. Somehow no woman was ever right for him. Unconsciously he longed for a mother goddess, a perfect mother who would cosset him, care for him and supply his every need. The greatest fear of the puer aeternus type of man is entrapment, because he is already caught in the mother complex itself. The one overwhelming desire in a confining situation is to escape from it. This form of neurosis has been described as the 'provisional life' which is an unfulfilled life because it is not yet. It is as if only the future holds the promise of the best of life. Thus, the man is always passively waiting.

The sudden blindness of the left eye occasioned by the retinal detachment and which coincided with the grave deterioration of the skin, was for him, a dire warning. The archetypal power was nearing explosive force. The skin had for years revealed a 'furor dermaticus' an inner rage of monumental proportion. Those aspects associated with the left eye, inner vision, passivity and the past were to be reviewed and understood. He was required to 'see' that is to understand the inner world of his emotionality, the cold and brutal shadow, with the distant inner anima figure. The sluggish nature of his responses to life and the chagrin engendered by the prison of his neurosis were to be rendered conscious and accepted.

The chance of freedom offered itself with the means to escape the strangulation of the mother-tie by way of understanding himself. Perhaps again the promise of the 'provisional life' beckoned, but the archetype waited no longer.

Before the chance to escape occurred, his heart failed him, and his escape came via another door. The deadly 'mother' as death claimed him.

The psychotherapist who was to work with him received a telephone call from the actual mother who said quite simply, "My son will not keep his appointment, he has died suddenly. It is for the best".

(4) THE HORSE BOY

A woman brought her son for therapy because it seemed he had developed an allergy to horses. He was eight years old, and every time he came into contact with horses he began to sneeze. This led to an eczematous reaction of the entire lower face. The mother of the boy was a woman who apparently knew the answer to almost everything. She had trained as a nurse, and was of the opinion that the real cause of her son's condition was the dander[14] of the horses. However skin tests had been found to be negative. The mother did not believe these results, and felt that somewhere a mistake had been made. She was sure that the horse had given the boy the allergy.

The reason for the concern was that the family, in the mother's words was 'mad about horses'. Since the boy had developed the allergy the activities of the family had been curtailed. The woman was extraordinarily concerned primarily because her elder daughter was an excellent horsewoman, and took part in a great number of horse trials and competitions. She was a star performer at these horse events, therefore it was imperative that the family supported her. It was quite clear that the mother was inordinately proud of her talented daughter.

During the mother's soliloquy the boy and I said not one word. It came to me however that it was not an allergy which had beset the boy but an antipathy. I felt uninclined to blame him for it. I asked the boy if he was afraid of horses. He admitted that he was afraid that they might kick him, but at once his mother intervened and pooh-poohed the statement with some asperity. The only solution, as far as I could see, was to repeat the tests, and try to reassure the mother should they prove to be negative. Indeed they did, so the task was to convince the mother that perhaps the cause of the problem lay elsewhere, and not with the horse.

I suggested to the boy that he might like to draw for me. He agreed at once, as did the mother but without enthusiasm. The drawing started and was accomplished with extraordinary zeal and outstanding verve. The mother said she was too busy to bring him regularly but would arrange that he was accompanied. The grandmother proved to be an admirable companion.

I was introduced over the weeks, to a mountain of drawings, every kind of animal was produced, wild, domesticated, rare, common, reptilian, mammalian, and also fish and birds. The detail was excellent, and the colours lively. Interestingly, and this was surprising, the original animals which he did belonged to the pre-historic age. Undoubtedly he had used a book in order to copy them, but it was of interest that the unconscious should choose just that period of pre-historic cave animals as an initiation.

Eventually he was to reach his 'horse period'. This was approximately two months or so after our first meeting. There were literally hundreds of horses. They occurred singly, in groups, sitting, lying, standing, running, or leaping. In every drawing there was a recurrent motif. In the right hand top corner, sometimes in the upper centre, there appeared a bright rayed sun always partially eclipsed by a cloud. Sometimes the sun's rays could be observed extending from behind the cloud as a kind of nimbus (pointing to its importance). When the horses appeared the sun, although still obscured, had emerged more fully from behind the cloud, as if the latter had slipped. Then followed a summation of the whole process.

He produced a series of drawings, five in all. The first was a dragon, which he described as a pre-historic Brontosaur (Greek Brontë = thunder, sauros = lizard). The sky above was blue-black without a sun. Then followed a horse and its foal. He explained it was a mare and her son. In the right hand top corner was the sun with its cloud. Then he showed me, with a face alight with joy, a wonderful drawing. He said 'You will like this!'. It was a large drawing of the skeleton of a horse. For so young a boy it was quite splendid. Moreover he had carefully copied out the name of every bone, tendon, muscle and organ of the horse. It was a perfect anatomical drawing.

When asked why he had drawn it, he replied that he had told his grandmother that one day he would do it. Then he borrowed his sister's horse book and he did it. The last drawing of all was again one of horses a mother and son, a mare and foal, standing in a meadow. Above from a clear blue sky the round orange globe of the sun, shone, without a cloud.

The boy and I got on very well. He was lively, intelligent, and a fine draughtsman. I asked few questions, other than those concerning certain points of the drawings. I did not draw attention to the clouded sun, I permitted the unconscious to speak through the pictures, without inteference on my part.

I was not surprised when the mother arrived to inform me that the boy was quite better and that horses no longer seemed to bother him. Both the boy and I were already aware of that fact. By drawing the skeleton of the horse, he had got to the 'bones' of his problem, and unconsciously he had dissected it anatomically.

The eczema was undoubtedly of atopic aetiology. He had an atopic diathesis, having suffered from dermatitis as a baby for a short period. It had been thought that the sneezing was due to the horse, but the problem was a psychological one.

A sneeze is a sudden involuntary and convulsive expulsion of air or breath through the nose or mouth. It is always accompanied by a characteristic sound. In the Heian period of Japanese history the courtiers of those days believed that a sneeze indicated a lie. The Greeks thought it prophetic, the voice of the soul, urging for expression.

What was expressed through the long continuous series of drawings was a stream of images reflecting a remarkable transformation of psychic energy. The boy did have a fear of the horse, which was unconscious, because repressed on account of his greater fear of his mother's derision. The transformation started at deep unconscious levels represented by the pre-historic cave animals. The animals themselves signified instinctual energy. At last the age of the mammal was reached. The motif of the cloud over the sun represented an over-riding unconsciousness of his own masculine consciousness, symbolized by the sun. The final summation series showed the total picture leading to the anatomical drawing. He handed them to me in the sequence he had draughted them. With this drawing, the fear of the horse was sacrificed, it was 'seen through'. Lastly again came the mare and the foal, and the cloud had disappeared, leaving the sun without impediment. Consciousness had integrated the unconscious problem, and the eczema and the sneezing both cleared never to recur.

The horse is a complex symbol because of its speed it signifies the light, and also fire, as well as the wind. There are the fiery horses of Helios, and the names of Hector's horses were Podargos which means swift of foot, Lampos, which is shining, Xanthos, yellow (the yellow sun of the drawings is recalled) and Aithon which means burning. The horse is often symbolized by the foam of sea water. It is therefore a symbol for energic forces. It is a warm blooded mammalian and represents instinct. Jung[15] has this to say about the horse, "It is man's steed and signifies a quantum of energy at man's disposal". He continues[16] "the libido directed towards the mother actually symbolizes her as a horse. The mother imago is a libido symbol, and so is the horse". The common factor in both is the libido, which according to Jung must be, as mother-libido sacrificed in order to create the world. The mother was a remarkably opinionated and managing woman. She was only concerned with the fact that her daughter was to shine at the horse events. She had not considered the individual nature of her son. First of all he was afraid of the horses, and secondly there was an element of jealousy of the sister. He had a good relationship with his grandmother who provided the constant support for him, which he lacked from his own mother. It was the fear of the latter which was the prime problem. On the surface, her acid tongue, but in the inner world it was the pull of the mother-libido. It was the latter which had to be overcome, the incest fear.

Because he was diligent, and liked to draw, he was able to introvert sufficiently so that his libido poured into the images. The sneezing and the facial eczema represented his outer inability to stand up to his mother, and inside, they represented the soul speaking. He was able eventually to throw off the maternal unconsciousness which impeded him in the form of his mother's negative attitude towards him. At last, ego consciousness asserted itself fully, in a positive discerning masculine way. This young person saw the goal, and aimed for it, which is the essence of masculinity.

This short series has been especially selected after a distillation of many hundreds of cases of atopic dermatitis. It is an endeavour to illustrate the powerful presence of the archetype of the mother, as it reveals itself in each instance. The essential problem is the disordered relationship between the mother and the child. The latter is the victim of its mother's neurosis. The advent of the child into the mother's life, appears to revivify and bring into focus, the negative aspect of the maternal archetype. All those childish fears, anxieties and neurotic traits of her own childhood are reactivated, and since unconscious become destructive. Until such time as the psychology of the parent is seriously considered, the disorder will continue to propagate itself into succeeding generations. The relationship between the mother and the unborn child during pregnancy and after its birth is of the utmost importance. The unconscious maternal reaction is the key upon which the future development of the child is dependent. If this knowledge can be introduced to the mother, enabling her to express any negativity, and if she is able to accept her deficiencies, there is reasonable hope of amelioration of the skin disorder for the offspring.

The unconscious psychic content in the mother-child bond is the archetype. Eczema is a superficial skin disorder of the epidermis, and the skin is the most superficial somatic organ. The essential nature of the primordial vesicle of the eczematous process is a volcano in miniature. If viewed as a symbol of unconscious psyche, eczema mirrors the immense energic urgency inherent in the archetype; and the immediacy of the potential for assimilation can be intuitively perceived.

It is remarkable how quickly the child's skin may reflect the mother's redemption by change of heart and attitude, induced by a recognition of the unconscious negativity which she holds against the child.

REFERENCES

1 Jung, C. G., Collected Works, Vol. 18, para 995, Routledge & Kegan Paul, London.
2 Ibid.
3 Von Franz, M-L., On Divination and Synchronicity, p. 100.
4 Jung, C. G., Collected Works, Vol. 5, para 460, Routledge & Kegan Paul, London.
5 Ibid., Vol. 12 para 32. Routledge & Kegan Paul, London.
6 Ibid., Vol. 9 11 para 60 Routledge & Kegan Paul, London.
7 Ibid.
8 Rook, A., Wilkinson, D. S., Ebling, F. J. G., Textbook of Dermatology, Blackwell, 1979, Atopic Dermatitis, Chapter 13.
9 Maguire, A., Psychic Possession Among Industrial Workers, The Lancet, 18 February 1978, p. 376–378.

10 Jung, C. G., Collected Works, Vol. 14, para 47, Routledge & Kegan Paul, London.

11 Layard, John, Making of Men in Malekula, p. 282, Eranos 1948.

12 Von Franz, M-L, Puer Aeternus, Sigo Press, 2nd Edition, p. 1. (from Ovid Metamorphoses iv 18–20).

13 Ibid.

14 Dander = dandruff or epidermal scales.

15 Jung, C. G., Collected Works, Vol. 5, para 421, Routledge & Kegan Paul, London.

16 Ibid., para 275, Routledge & Kegan Paul, London.

5

URTICARIA

A great many provoking causes are listed for this disorder, which is sometimes called nettle rash or hives. They include, foods, skin contacts, inhalants, drugs, infections, some general medical disorders as well as psychological factors. Furthermore the clinical features and the natural history are as varied and unpredictable as the aetiology. It has been said[1] "the establishment of the cause (of urticaria) is difficult and often impossible".

The truth of this statement was proved incontestably many years ago for me, during my training as a dermatologist. It was my task at that time to be responsible for an urticarial clinic which had been established for several decades. During the course of this work I dealt with thousands of cases. Because of my traditional medical training I firmly believed in those days that with a fully comprehensive scientific investigation accompanied by goodwill on the part of the subject, the cause could be discovered. Some of the sufferers had histories extending over several decades. Since I worked in a prestigious medical centre, and was possessed of immense enthusiasm, there was no difficulty in setting up the researches. Every patient who attended that clinic was subjected to a full investigation of every aspect of the physical being. The sad outcome over a period of three years was that I was not one whit the wiser as to the individual physical cause. However a curious experience occurred towards the end of the investigative period. I myself, developed an acute attack of urticaria of the hands. Needless to say I was horrified, for the prospect of several years of the disorder was not enticing. I was about to investigate myself when quite by chance, I was delivered of a most singular intuitive thought. I realized that in my own case, the condition was due to the fact that I had refused to acknowledge consciously that I was possessed of a brooding resentment, which had developed over a period of weeks. The moment I consciously accepted my emotion, and dealt with it, the urticaria vanished. I had been as it were, immersed in urticaria, and this revelation can only be described as an act of divine grace. From that moment, I relinquished all scientific investigative aims, and began to talk to the patients about their inner emotional lives. I made a point of enquiring the precise date of the onset of the condition, and the circumstances surrounding its debut. At first this was difficult but with persistence the fact became clear that the state of the emotional life of the patient when the urticaria developed was of vital importance. The aim was to retrieve it and encourage the subject to become conscious of it, and retain it in consciousness.

The symptom apart from the eruption itself which urges the patient to seek therapy is irritation. Sometimes it is described as burning in nature or even stinging. Usually it is excruciatingly severe and may be described as a "furor dermaticus". The appearances of the ephemeral red patches accompanied by raised welts exhibits constant change, as first one site and then another is affected. The actual diagnosis of such a characteristically changing pattern is relatively easy. The need to scratch produces an inflammatory reaction which reaches its peak fairly quickly then slowly subsides, to disappear practically without trace, only to reappear in a different site. One is reminded of a heath fire, which smoulders then blazes forth with an intense heat, only to die down and later strike up again in another distant venue.

Scratching is constant, and sometimes a savage fury can be discerned as the finger nails claw unremittingly at the skin; misery and dejection are co-partners. Yet, bearing in mind the physical presence of these factors one is frequently surprised to find that the demeanour of the subject is curiously detached, in that there appears to be a calm acceptance unrelated to the actual fiery appearance of the skin.

A psychological assessment of such persons who develop urticaria reveals a willingness to serve. Nothing is too much trouble in their efforts to aid and be of help to others. They tend to overload themselves with an onerous burden of duties, even to the point of martyrdom. In most instances, the cardinal sin is against inner instinctual nature, and the body via the skin indicates its grave displeasure in the form of a fiery eruption. In observing the skin objectively, the conclusion cannot be avoided that above all other dermatoses, urticated skin reflects the inner emotional psychic life. Indeed it becomes a looking glass into the inner world, where resentment, brooding anger, murderous rage, and almighty wrath becomes visible. In the hidden darkness of a personality which holds itself too light or too pure, a conflict has occurred, which can only be resolved by the conscious acceptance of certain unconscious contents. The changeable and ephemeral nature of the urticarial reaction, dependent upon underlying vascular change, reveals the relative superficiality of those self-same contents and indicates the possibility of their integration into consciousness.

In conclusion the appearance of urticaria is a statement of the shadow. This is the name given by Jung to the archetype that represents one's gender, and influences a person's relations with his own sex. Since the shadow has historically very deep roots, it is the most powerful and probably (in potentia) the most dangerous of all archetypes. It contains much of man's basic animal nature, which in the course of the civilizing process becomes suppressed. Thus he becomes alienated from his inner instinctual nature and loses contact with its wisdom. An individual without a shadow is superficial and lacking in depth of spirit, since he has lost the realm of insights spontaneous creativity and deep strong emotions. Allenby[2] quoting Jung, said "Our unconscious energies give momentum to our journey through life and if we direct their course, our actions will have strength, we may even sense that God is behind us".

If however we omit to do so the continually active energies do not receive form or direction in consciousness. Then the way is paved for the subject to be victimized by his unconscious needs and desires.

Often it seems that the urticarial response issues directly from a specific cause, such as an allergy to shell-fish, or roses, or perfume, penicillin or human maternal milk, on the one hand, whilst on the other, an adverse contact with the elements, such as heat, cold, water, or the sun. However it is wise always to consider the psychic situation in order to ascertain the meaning inherent in the reaction.

A young woman was referred with a severe solar urticaria. She was of outstanding beauty, but came from comparatively humble circumstances. She came in great distress because her life had become intolerable, each time she went into sunlight she developed a fierce urticarial reaction. She was investigated at various institutions specializing in this condition, and eventually she was told that the only solution was to avoid sunlight.

The cause seemed to be clear, she had in simple terms an allergy to the sun, or indeed one might say an antipathy. Consciously this was not the case. The story which unfolded as she revealed her distress, was that she had become the mistress of an extremely rich man. His pastime was to sail an ocean going yacht in the southern tropical seas, and he liked her to join him whenever possible, which was in fact fairly frequently. In these circumstances she was exposed directly to the ultraviolet light from the sun, and also in the reflected light from the ocean. Her solar exposure was total. The woman had a husband, and a small child of three or four years, in order to join her lover she left them both for long periods. Thus her duties and responsibilities as wife and mother were disregarded, and eventually neglected. She badly wanted to divorce her husband and marry the man, but the latter who was also married refused. Since she was unable to make up her mind it seemed that the unconscious did it for her. Here was a woman seduced by materialism, and severed from her instinctual nature.

She was deeply unconscious of herself and had no conception of her self-ish, deceitful and coldly cruel shadow, nor of the sufferings caused to her husband and child. Neither was she conscious of the true nature of her lover. She was eventually forced into darkness out of the blinding burning rays of the sun, forced it would seem, to persuade her to realize her own dark nature. This was the meaning inherent in the solar urticaria. She was undoubtedly allergic to the light of day.

The following cases of urticaria reveal the role of the unconscious in each particular instance as it intrudes into an individual life, victimizes it, and forces it to a higher level of conscious awareness.

SERPENT GIRL

Many years ago, a general practitioner telephoned me and asked if I would see as an urgent case a young woman who was quite seriously ill. She had become ill several weeks earlier, with a progressively severe cholinergic urticaria, with spasmodic bouts of angio-neurotic oedema. The doctor was of the opinion that these attacks were endangering her life. She had always been of good health, and had not previously suffered from any skin allergy but she had recently bought a snake, and the doctor thought perhaps that she was allergic to the snake; in fact he was convinced that it was the snake which was causative as she had bought it the day before the so called allergy had started.

The young woman was quite presentable, she was twenty-five years of age, and was a school teacher. She lived with her parents, and had only ever been away from her home for a period of two years at a teachers' training college. After she had qualified as a junior school mistress she returned to her home, and got a job at a school in her home town, where she had been born and brought up.

The urticaria had appeared six weeks earlier, and exactly as the doctor had said, on the day following the purchase of a snake. She told me that she hoped it was not an allergy as she liked the snake and wanted to keep it, it was a non-poisonous green grass snake. She volunteered the information that she kept it under her bed, and fed it each day with warm milk.

The most significant part of the history as far as I could judge at that time was the acquisition of such an extraordinary purchase, by a young adult woman of twenty-five years. When asked why she had bought such a creature, she said "because it is clean, quiet and causes no trouble at home". In fact that sentence was the most telling, because she was in describing the snake, describing her own self, it was in effect the story of her life.

In the subsequent discussion which I had with her, it came to light that a week before the advent of the snake, the young woman had been very distressed. One evening she had gone out with her fiancée, whom she had met some two years previously, becoming engaged to him the following year. At the end of the evening, he had quite suddenly, without a quarrel, and certainly without any preamble, broken off the engagement. The young woman was apparently very distressed but since the fiancée had decided not to discuss the matter, the painful conversation so described had quickly terminated the friendship. On arrival at her home, she told her mother of her distress, and her mother's reply was quite simply, a non-commital shrug of the shoulders without an immediate riposte. Then the mother told her that it was a good thing that the engagement had been broken off, and that she would now get someone who was better, with a better job, and with more money.

After this the girl described to me that she had gone at once to her bedroom, where she had remained for a whole week. She saw no one except her parents, and she did nothing, except sleep and stare at the bedroom walls. At the end of the week, she got up, and went out for a walk, during which she passed a pet shop. Whilst gazing into the window of the latter, her eye alighted upon a green snake. She entered the shop and purchased the creature. She then returned to her bedroom, and put it under the bed, and fed it with saucers of milk.

When asked why she had not bought a puppy or a kitten she said that she dared not, as her mother had a beautiful house, and would not allow an animal, because it might ruin the furniture. In all her life the young woman had never been allowed to possess a pet of any description, because of the mother's embargo.

I asked her if she was angry with the young man for breaking off the engagement, and in doing so in such a peremptory way. She looked quite startled and answered that she was not. She then told me that her mother had told her after the rupture that she would never make a good wife for a man, and she believed that her mother was right. I then asked her if she was perhaps angry with her mother. Again she shook her head, but then she became very upset, and told me that she was amazed that I would ask such a question. Shortly afterwards she expressed the desire to leave and I terminated the examination, and she went home. I did not expect to see her again as I felt my last question had shocked her profoundly. Her expression as she left was one of cold fury directed towards me.

Six weeks later however she returned to see me, alert, happy and cured, in that the urticaria had resolved itself without any therapy from me. She explained that she had not intended to return to see me, as my question about her mother had both shocked her and angered her deeply. She was angry with me because I had upset her with a personal and uninvited question. When she arrived home she became very depressed again. However she did not retire to her bed, as she had done on the previous occasion of the depression which had arisen from the severance of the engagement. Slowly she came to realize that she hated her fiancée but also her mother who had seemed pleased about the fact of her unhappiness. She also remembered that her mother had never allowed her to do anything she wanted to do, she even became a teacher because it was her mother's plan. The fiancée, she believed had treated her exactly as had her mother, in that he decided where they would go and what they would do. She had always pleasantly agreed to his plans without demur.

Suddenly in the middle of her discourse, she said to me 'Do you know why I bought the snake?' She answered herself, 'I bought it because it looks exactly like mother'.

This girl's story revealed how the unconscious had concretized the mother's cold repellant attitude. The girl had never consciously registered the mother's coldness, nor had she realized the exertion of power on the mother's part. The girl herself had an extraverted attitude, and feeling was her superior function. For almost twenty years this young woman had believed her mother to be related and warm, she knew that her mother was very proud of her house, and fastidious to the point of obsession regarding its upkeep, but she had not realized that in fact the house was more important than she was. Certainly this young woman believed or forced herself to believe that she loved her mother unreservedly. She was not aware nor did she permit herself to be conscious of the fact that she bore an unconscious resentment towards he mother because of the latter's obsessive attitudes, unrelatedness, and coldness.

It was interesting that it was a grass snake, this is the healing serpent of the god Apollo, the divine healer, and his son, Asklepios, the deity of the physicians. When she thought the snake looked like her mother, it was because the snake symbolized the unrelated feeling. There was indeed without doubt an unrelated Eros on the part of the mother but also a projection on the part of the patient. Projection is based upon the archaic identity of subject and object but the term is used only when the necessity has already arisen which demands resolution of the identity with the object.

A further word regarding projection may be helpful. It was first used by Sigmund Freud who believed projection to be a defence mechanism through which a neurotic person freed himself of a feeling of conflict. The feeling held by the subject was displaced onto another as the intended object. Jung also used the term, but because of his different view of the unconscious he gave it a new interpretation. Jung described projection as an unconscious automatic process, that is a process which is not perceived by the subject and is not intentional, whereby psychic contents or a certain psychic content transfers itself to an object, and appears to belong to that object. "The projection ceases the moment it becomes conscious, that is to say when it is seen to belong to the subject."[3] Jung emphasised that projection is "never conscious, projections are always there first, and recognised afterwards."[4]

The snake symbolized the reality of the unrelated feeling on the part of the mother and also the unrelatedness of the mother complex itself as well as the unexpressed hostility on the part of the girl. At the same time however it was for her, a symbol of healing.

In the subsequent six weeks after her first visit for the skin condition, she had become conscious of the fact that she was angry with the fiancée, and more importantly with her mother. This brought release, and healing. She was then able to make a decision to leave home, acquire an apartment for herself, which she also furnished with a puppy as a pet, instead of the snake, which she eventually relinquished. The acquisition of the snake was the first act of defiance in twenty-five years.

The mother's destructive animus which spoke so clearly on the fateful night of the broken engagement was so to speak an unrelated snake, perceived in the cold inhuman attack without provocation which was made upon her daughter. The animosity was also substantiated in the opinionated views, quite without foundation which were held by the mother regarding the suitability of her daughter as a wife. It was the animus which the girl had re-visualized in a fleeting instant in the hypnotic eye of the snake, a reptile far far removed from human consciousness in the time scale of its ancient lineage. The skin disease, urticaria, was for this girl symbolic of the casting of the snake's skin, and was a forerunner to a rebirth, and a new level of consciousness and adaptation.

Urticaria is an exceedingly commonplace disorder, and most people at one time or another suffer from this malady. As has been earlier stated, it is usually regarded as an allergy to something or other, albeit the allergen is rarely pin pointed or isolated. During the years of my own practice as both dermatologist and analyst, as also stated, I found that urticaria represents unexpressed emotionality, the emotion which is usually foremost is that of anger.

The most striking feature of this case was the fact that a young woman suddenly after a period of depression following the break-up of a romantic attachment, purchased a green grass snake. One must enquire of oneself in such a circumstance, what is the meaning of such an act? What was the intention of psyche, in inducing a thoroughly modern young person living in an urban community to do such a thing? For most people snakes are held in a kind of awe, for many they are regarded with terror, but for all there is usually attached an element of fear, either conscious or unconscious.

The acquisition of a harmless green grass snake, represented something quite vast and invisible. For into this girl's life there had emerged the archeypt of the serpent. This had probably been constellated during the week long incubation period in her bedroom. The skin disease which itself was to symbolize a rebirth into a new attitude came at exactly the moment the girl bought the snake. The inner and outer events revealed the synchronicity and the presence of the archetype.

Jung[5] explains that the synchronicity principle asserts that the terms of a meaningful coincidence are connected by simultaneity and meaning. In his paper on synchronicity he states that synchronistic events are "acts of creation and that way they are unique. They are also so exceptional that most people doubt their existence."[6]

It would seem that the severance of the bond between the young woman and her fiancée brought on the depression, altogether natural in the circumstances, which was a reflection of unconscious unexpressed anger. The return of the energic value of the relationship to the unconscious during the period of deep introversion in her bedroom appears to have activated the archetype of the serpent, the archetype of disease and healing. The quantum of libido freed by the break-down of the relationship, was available because the girl had had real feeling for the fiancée. It was this libido originally, which the fiancée had managed to steal away from the mother complex, and when it was discarded by his cruel rejection, it became free again for the next step. Her healing began in the seclusion of her room and the deep introversion allowed healing to proceed at this deep archetypal level. Although the powerful mother complex remained, its gripping power was being depotentiated during that vital week, because she was already rising to a higher level of consciousness, and had realized, her own hostility.

In order to look for a moment at the meaning of the serpent-archetype, it is useful to remember at this point that the actual physical body of the snake combines the motility of the animal in its displacements and the spiral process of vegetal life in its innate actual muscular reflex movements. It is this strange combination which grips and fascinates this combination of opposites of both animal and plant attributes, the utter stillness, and the lightning speed of its movements. The essence of the hypnotic effect is found in the snake's unblinking glittering regard and the rapidly constantly darting tongue.

In Hellenic mythology the healing aspect first associated with the snake was contained in the oracular crevice at Delphi, in all the temples devoted to Hermes, Asklepios, and later Mithra. In these temples there was always a cave, grotto or well, and the chthonic god who inhabited these sites and who had to be placated with gifts, since he represented the earth itself, as a devouring mother, was usually a snake.

That the snake is really a death symbol is found in the fact that the souls of the dead like the chthonic gods appear as serpents and dwellers in the kingdom of the deadly mother. In Ancient Greece the caduceus of the god of the physicians Asklepios was a staff with one serpent wound round it. Five centuries before Christ temples were built to this greatly revered god at Cos, Epidauros, Pergamum and Athens. Each temple, or Asklepieion contained a central place which housed the temple snake which was fed on milk and honey and which was also the god, Asklepios in his snake form, for he was both the snake, and the god. In the temenos of the temple, in the spellbinding centre, pilgrims came to worship the god, by bathing, and prayers then they lay down to sleep and to await a dream, in which the god in the form of a man or a snake, would visit them and bring the healing. The period of waiting was called the incubatio, and was exactly such a period as our young woman teacher experienced prior to her rising from her bed to go out and at once, purchase a snake. There is little doubt that in that time of darkness and depression the girl was visited by the god of healing himself, and the image which she bore unconsciously, presented itself to her in reality in the god's serpentine form, when she began to recover.

The serpent archetype, the archetype of constant renewal and rebirth is represented by the image of the reptile which sheds its skin and is reborn as a new and shiny being, and as such symbolizes a transformation from illness to health, and new life. Psychologically the light of consciousness is born, and there is a dawning of awareness, this realization brings relief of symptoms and eventual healing. And so it was with the school teacher.

I did little for this girl, I asked simply a question, after she had begun to experience the healing process. I always felt with this particular patient, that I had been given a truly immense gift. I was allowed to witness personally a transformation from sickness to health, and I learned from this experience that the urticarial reaction occurs when ego consciousness is capable at last of accepting unconscious contents. Contents which have risen and reached the zonal area which marks the boundary between consciousness and the personal unconscious. In other words, they are contents which can be accepted. Whether they are or not depends on many factors, but the most important is that the patient has a guide either in the inner or outer world. In this case, the young woman received the guidance of an inner psychopompos, and the synchronicity occasioned by the archetype, included my own observations.

THE STRAWBERRY MAN

About a quarter of a century ago, at the time of the world crisis occasioned by the conflict between the United States and the Union of Soviet Russia which came to a head in the geographical situation known as the Bay of Pigs, a man in his middle fifties was referred with chronic urticaria.

He had suffered from distressing attacks over a period of several months, and he had come to the conclusion that he was allergic to strawberries. This was proved by the fact, according to his own observations, that he usually though not always had an attack after he had partaken of these delectable fruits. He was a journalist, and as a foreign correspondent, for a prestigious newspaper he was a man well known in the world of the press, being a leading expert upon current affairs. Because of the crisis in the Caribbean, he had been posted to Mexico, and had perforce to cross the Atlantic ocean several times a month in order to discourse with the editorial staff of his newspaper. It was during these transatlantic air trips in which he always travelled as a first class passenger that he was able to enjoy strawberries, of which he was apparently very fond.

The diagnosis proved to be urticaria, and all the tests proved that his health was excellent, without any physical abnormalities. During consultations it became apparent that the urticaria only developed when he ate strawberries on a flight from Mexico City to Europe, surprisingly not when he flew in the reverse direction. This information came to light after he had been asked as to why he continued to eat the fruit when he knew he might have a such sharp reaction. Indeed just such an attack, had been observed personally at the beginning when his face was swollen his eyes semi-closed, and he was scratching furiously because of the generalised irritation occasioned by the condition.

He later divulged that his life had taken on a rather erratic nature because of the crisis and although he still lived in Europe, he had to be based in Central America, even so he had also to fly a good deal between Central and South America. On his visits to Europe, he visited 'his editor and then his wife'. He made the flat statement in just that order. In his own words he had become rootless, and wondered if perhaps stress was causative of his condition.

He came several times, and each occasion provided a sight of a classical urticarial reaction. He then gave up eating strawberries altogether, but to his great disappointment he continued to develop urticaria each time he came to Europe. He then began to wonder if perhaps something else was the cause. When asked about his life, he said that he had been married thirty years, but only his wife was at home, the children having gone their various ways. It was pointed out to him the strange fact that the eruption always appeared when he came home. He did not take the point.

About this time, when he had discussed his family life and the fact that he liked Mexico City very much, I myself happened to go to the cinema one evening following a consultation with him to see an Ingmar Bergman's film called 'Wild Strawberries'. The haunting film was full of pretty young women, all indeed of a fragile blond beauty, seemingly eternally young, and who were undoubtedly all anima figures. I was oddly perturbed by the old professor's dream-like reflections and I became aware of the 'defendu' quality of the wild strawberry-gathering in the woods with its associations of youth and fleeting and transient romantic summer love, so soon to disappear and perhaps die. With it there was also a distinctly erotic aspect which underlay the extraordinary fragile and tender quality of the relationships.

The strawberry is the attribute of certain love goddesses because it is cool and dry when greenish white in colour, and deep red, moist, and sweet, when ripe. It is sometimes used as a medicinal talisman and in Bavaria it used to be the custom to leave strawberries out in early summer for the elves in order to guarantee prosperity and fertility in the home. It is in Christianity an emblem of John the Baptist, and also the Virgin Mary, but much earlier in pagan times the strawberry was the attribute of the Nordic goddess Frigga who presided over marriages. It was said that on St. John's Day, the summer equinox of June 24th that she would go in search of wild strawberries with the children as later would the Virgin. It was also believed that on that day no mother who had lost a little child must taste a strawberry as it was a forbidden fruit. If she did her little child would get none in Heaven for the Virgin would say "You must stand aside for your mother has already eaten your share, and none remains for you".[7] (There is evidence here of an intrusion of Christian morality replacing the former paganism.)

On the other side of the world, the strawberry has a particular significance amongst the Ojibwa Indians,[8] in the South West of Ontario in Canada. When a man died his soul which remained conscious on going towards the land of the dead, came at last upon an enormous strawberry. For the Indians, the strawberry was the food of summer and symbolized the good season. If the soul of the dead man tasted this strawberry, he would forget the world of the living, and all return to life and the land of the living would for him become impossible. If however he refused to touch the strawberry he would have the possibility of returning to earth. As with Persephone, earthly nourishment is forbidden to the inhabitants of the underworld.

The following week the patient reappeared and at the moment of his entrance into my prescence I had a sudden memory image of the film. The strawberries which he had eaten were not wild strawberries but were most certainly out of season. In fact that is exactly how he described them to me on the occasion of his first visit.

Here was a lively intelligent and attractive man in full middle age, secure in a marriage of three decades, a marriage both solid and reassuring. In his transportation to Central America he had not only been removed to the new centre of action but he had become separated from his former life, albeit temporarily.

He spoke throughout of Mexico City in the most glowing terms, he conjured up a city of immense vitality and beauty, features which cannot be denied. The tones of his description went further than those usually given in the normal course of events, and it became clear that Mexico City was to be understood as something else. The attraction of that city began to take the form of a woman. I asked him directly about the marriage and whether there was someone else. He gave me a long slow reflective look, and dropped his eyes for a full minute, he then looked directly at me and assured me that all was well with his wife. In that glance he revealed that he knew at once that the psychological conflict occasioned by the love of two women, stood solidly behind the development of urticaria.

In finding this new love he had lost himself, for it had come to possess him, and unconsciously his marriage and old wife of thirty years had become irksome, and resentment had begun to build up. This was quite unconscious, but the regular appearance of the skin eruption, during the journey home to his domestic hearth was an expression of the exacerbation of this resentment each time. It seemed on the surface as if the strawberry was the cause, but the strawberry itself was incidental, it was all that which the strawberry symbolized in his unconscious psyche, wherein lay the difficulty.

Although there were deep resentments against the shackles of the marriage, not a trace of opprobrium appeared when discussing it. He had completely partitioned off the two aspects of his life, the masculine world of his newspaper which included, although on the boundary his home and wife, and the new exciting and ostensibly Christian Mexico City, with its overwhelming pagan overtones. It was from underneath the Zocalo in front of the modern cathedral in that city in 1824 that the monstrous sculpture of Coatlicue, the Earth Goddess of the Aztecs was discovered. She was worshipped there in the ancient Aztec capital of Tenochtitlan from whose ruins Mexico City itself arose. The figure of the goddess is horrifying to European eyes, used to the sweet gentle gaze of the Virgin, but to the Aztecs she represents the Earth itself and the statue is a poem in thanksgiving for her pain and her generosity in giving food and life to mankind. She more than anything else expresses the dynamism and abundance of the feminine and in particular of maternal nature in that vast region.

This city was to be the cradle of the new feminine attachment of the journalist, this love was a secret in reality even to himself. He had to face consciously the conflict with its delights and its resentments, he had to become aware of the opposites in himself and he had to face his own inner nature. The Self sent to him via the humble skin disorder of urticaria the means whereby he was to return to his own reality, and become conscious of his situation, and that of the two women, unknown to each other, unaware of each other who were both equal partners in the conflict. The skin disease was to 'earth' him.

The secret had to be exposed and integrated into consciousness and so the strawberry proved to be a most significant symbol, for the irritation and the suffering caused by the urticaria was a forward step in his individuation process, coming to consciousness of self.

The strawberry with all its connotations of eroticism, youth and fleeting beauty, sweet ripeness and marriage but also for its caché or 'defendu' quality was the perfect symbol which ushered his plunge into a bed of nettles. Nettle rash is the common name for urticaria. A nettle is a plant of the genus Urtica of which the species Urtica Dioica, the common or great nettle and Urtica Urens, the small nettle grow profusely on waste land and waysides, especially if untrodden. They are covered with stinging hairs which produce through their histaminic effect an urticarial rash or nettle rash. With distinctive epithets the name of nettle is given to a number of plants belonging to other genera, as blind deaf dead red or white nettles.

The archetype of the anima is that which leads a man into relationships and into life. The archetype is represented by a feminine image which represents for a man his fate. The anima herself led our patient into a conflict, in miniature which only he could solve. A conflict played out against the background of momentous events taking place in the political history of the world. For him the urticaria was the outward manifestation of the inner unconscious rage and resentment against the marriage tie. The cure lay in the conscious realization that his real problem was not a dermatological disorder but a psychic conflict. The strawberry urticaria, and the secret love conflict exhibited the phenomenon of synchronicity, the fiery outer eruption was the other face of the inner turmoil of the soul.

THE MAN WITH THE DOMINATING MOTHER

The case to be described has been chosen for the startling suddenness of the amelioration of symptoms after only one consultation. The patient was a thin anxious man, rather tall, but with a kyphosis which made him appear shorter than he actually was. He had a bright face, and an alert expression, but the anxious demeanour gave him the air of someone who was heavily burdened. He was referred by his doctor with an attack of giant urticaria which was totally disabling. The attack had begun two weeks previously and had reached a crescendo two or three days prior to his consultation. He was in a state of terror. The reason for this was that forty years previously at the age of twenty-seven he had had a previous attack which had persisted for twenty years without remission. During those twenty years he had suffered severely and the two decades of torture had imprinted themselves upon his mind. Psychologically one is permitted to say that he had an urticaria complex.

The story which unfolded was that he had lost his father when he was a boy, and he had been brought up by his mother. At the age of twenty-seven he became engaged to be married, and was in fact still living at home with his mother, at the time. Prior to the engagement he had tried on two separate occasions to leave England and go to work in the Far East, in a clerical capacity. Each time that he made an application to venture forth his mother had obstructed him, so in the end he gave up all notion of leaving England, and relinquished his dream. Then one afternoon shortly after becoming engaged and during the course of a tennis match the urticaria had started. It was a hot afternoon, and at first he thought he had 'heat lumps' a common term applied to urticaria. The interesting fact is that just before the ill-omened tennis match he had, on account of his fiancée's encouragement applied once again for a post in the Far East and on this occasion, without his mother's knowledge, and consequently without her obstruction, he was successful.

As soon as he received confirmation he told his mother of his plans and a most serious quarrel ensued. For the next twelve days his mother did not address one word to him. During this period he became increasingly distressed, and decided after discussing the matter with his fiancée not to go to the Far East. He then after the decision had been made, applied his mind as to how he could placate his mother.

He had saved some money by doing extra work in the evenings, so he decided to go to the bank and withdraw it. The money had been part of a reserve fund for his future marriage. The present which he bought for his mother was a candlestick made of twisted cut glass. He said he bought it to coax her out of her mood, and to forgive him for disobeying her!

After this quarrel the patient's prospective father-in-law died, and he was invited to take over the family business. This he did, and as he was successful, he became a reasonably well off man. He then stayed in the town of his birth for the rest of his life.

The day that he bought the placatory gift for his mother was the day of the tennis match, and the urticarial rash began on the back. From the moment of its onset there was no respite for twenty years, until quite suddenly from one day to the next it disappeared as he put it 'without any reason'. During the two decades in which he suffered the disorder he married, and he and his wife brought up their family. He said that he had visited 'hundreds of doctors', and was told that he had allergies to house dust, dust mites, pollen, fungal spores dry rot spores, cat dander, and so on. No cure was found for him, until the day it disappeared by itself. Then he forgot all about it, until exactly twenty years later when it returned just as before and with great severity. He had three children, a son who had become an architect, and two daughters whom he described as gipsies. When asked to elaborate upon this description he said they were 'foot-loose' travellers, one was in South America, travelling constantly, and the other was in Europe likewise constantly travelling from place to place. He was only able to describe their jobs rather scantily, but the loose term of hotel business seemed to cover their activities.

When asked what exactly had triggered off the present episode he answered without the trace of hesitation and explained that it was during the party for his mother's ninetieth birthday. It seemed that his wife had arranged the party and she had asked an old friend, a lady of eighty years to be a guest, as a companion as it were, for the aged parent, who it seemed had no friends left of her own age. The old mother took great exception to the proposed presence of the newcomer and would not allow her to attend the party, which consisted solely of the family, since she would not permit outsiders. During the party the patient began to feel unwell and he noticed that an urticarial rash had appeared on his hands and arms, which was intensely irritating. Before very long, and certainly before the end of the party he realized that his whole body was affected, and with this knowledge he was seized by the monstrous thought that it might last as before, for twenty years.

On the occasion of that first visit, after he had told the story as it is written he enquired just what the allergy might be. It was explained to him quite succinctly that undoubtedly he had only one real allergy and it was to his mother. At this, he suddenly stood up, he had been in a hunched crouching position leaning forward in the chair towards me. He exclaimed "that's right, that's it, I always knew it". The expression upon his face was one of intense suffering. He had always known that his mother was the great problem of his life, but he had never allowed himself to believe it. At the moment of confrontation with the actuality of the situation, he could accept it, at the age of sixty-seven years.

When he returned some weeks later it was to reveal that the eruption had cleared at once, not to return. He also made an interesting observation. He said that the discussion at the party had centred round the question as to whether or not Britain should remain as a member of the European Common Market. Suddenly his mother expressed the view that she sincerely hoped that Britain would withdraw as she had never had a decent orange to eat, since Britain had joined. The patient added that, at that moment the eruption began. He had decided, that his mother was a narrow-minded, opinionated old woman, and furthermore had always been so. But this realization however only, came, after reflection upon the medical discussion.

This case history depicts a tremendously crippling mother complex, which had held sway until the seventh decade of a man's life. Albeit, although it seemed he had escaped from it when he became affianced to his future wife, he was in fact still possessed. This was evidenced by his feeble capitulation at the first sign of his mother's displeasure after his third attempt to flee to the Far East. He was caught not only by the outer mother, but also by the inner internalised mother. It is interesting that after two decades of suffering, when the children began to leave home, and incidentally the grandmother's jurisdiction, the urticaria disappeared. It was also the time when he felt liberated and he explained that for the first time he and his wife felt that they were free to please themselves. Then suddenly after twenty years of freedom from irritation like a thunder-clap it returned, when his mother brought up the subject of the orange.

The orange is regarded as being of a celestial nature, it is the colour of the sun, and it is symbolic of the feminine principle, since it signifies fecundity. In the Far East it is given to a young girl when an offer of marriage is to be made, because it is reputed to come from the timeless tree, and as such is a bringer of good fortune, and immortality. In ancient English folk lore, it used to play a nefarious role in witchcraft, when it symbolized a victim's heart. The victim's name was written on a piece of paper, and then stuck on the orange which was placed high in the chimney where it remained until the victim died. The fact that the mother had a great propensity to wound to isolate, and to retreat into silence in order to punish, indicates her witch-like character revealed to her son, her mean-spirited narrowness of outlook, and that was the moment the urticaria returned. In retrospect it was the vital thought which led him to recovery, after all those years, in an instant he really understood the nature of his mother's bigoted animus for the first time, and so he was released, by illumination.

The disorder had begun forty years earlier at a tennis match. The symbolism of a tennis match is important. A game is fundamentally a struggle either against one's own weakness, doubt, or fear, or perhaps against the elements, hostile forces or death. One is reminded of the ball games of the Lakota, the Plains Indians of North America known commonly as Teton or Western Sioux. One of the seven sacred rites of the Teton which means snake, was to throw the ball, it was called Tapa Wankayeyapi, which means 'throwing the ball upwards'. The ball on being thrown by a young girl was caught, and the winner considered himself fortunate because the ball was symbolically equated with knowledge.

In the language of symbolism the ball represents a quantum of energy. In the tennis match our patient was suffering the internal conflict engendered by his mother's displeasure. The question was how could he placate her? It was a question which remained unanswered until the truth was realized four decades later, and by then there was no longer a necessity to placate, for the neurosis was over at last.

By refusing to live his life as a voyager or traveller, it was left for his daughters to live that part of his unlived life for him, and become gipsies.

REFERENCES

1 Rook, A., Wilkinson, D. S. Ebling, F. J. G., Textbook of Dermatology, Vol. 1, p. 974 3rd Edition, Blackwell Scientific Publications.
2 Jung, C. G., C. G. Jung Speaking, Allenby, p. 158 Ed. Wm. McGuire & R. F. C. Hill, Oxford.
3 Jung, C. G., Collected Works, Vol. 9, 1 p. 121, Routledge & Kegan Paul, London.
4 Ibid., p. 122.
5 Jung, C. G., Collected Works, Vol. 8, p. 916, Routledge & Kegan Paul, London.
6 Jung, C. G., Collected Works, Vol. 8, p. 938, Routledge & Kegan Paul, London.
7 Friend, H., Flowers and Flower Lore, Vol. 1, p. 107.
8 Servier, J. L'Homme et L'Invisible, 1964, p. 18.

6

PSORIASIS

This is a common skin disorder which usually presents without symptoms. It is occasionally accompanied by irritation and sometimes pain. The essential lesion is a raised red plaque covered with silvery scales. These plaques may be present anywhere on the body but particularly at sites subjected to repeated traumata. Very often, psoriasis is found on the scalp where it may have existed for several years mistakenly thought to be a severe dandruff, likewise it can affect the perianal areas unbeknown to the sufferer. It may also affect the entire body including the finger and toe nails. The condition gives rise to feelings of uncleanness, and even shame in the subject, because of its nature, and the fact that there is a constant shedding of scales.

THE PSORIATIC LESION.

The advent of the electron microscope has brought a vast increase of information concerning the cellular structure of the skin of the human embryo. It is therefore helpful to examine the structure of the latter.

When the foetal heart starts to beat at the end of the third week of intrauterine life, the epidermis consists of only one layer of cells. Three weeks later there are two layers, the outer periderm, and the inner germinal or basal layer. At sixteen weeks one or more intermediate layers have developed and by the age of twenty-six weeks, the periderm cells separate off, and the epidermis develops its mature form of four or five layers as is found in the adult skin. The innermost layer or basal layer is composed of cells which parent the other layers. The outermost layer is the most superficial and is called the keratin (horny) layer. This is the one which can be seen, and touched in the adult.

With the development of the horny layer, the human foetus has reached the reptilian stage of development.[1] The keratin layer begins its long history in the amphibia as a single layer, but in the human being it consists of fine keratin plaques or squames. In the reptile world, this layer is of the greatest importance, where it is characterized by thick, horny, epidermal scales, which usually overlap each other. In the crocodile and soft skin of the tortoise, keratin is shed continuously in small flakes (in much the same way as in that of the normal human being). In lizards and snakes, there is intermittent epidermal growth and keratinization, which results in periodic sloughing of the whole horny layer, a process designated as skin casting. A fission layer of unkeratinized cells separates the old from the newly formed scale. Normally not more than two generations of cells of the horny layer are present at any one time. Scales similar to those of the reptile are also found on the feet of birds, and the tails of some mammals, but the cells retain their nuclei.

This is comparable to the parakeratotic layer of the human psoriatic plaque, the essential lesion of the human dermatosis, psoriasis.

The silvery scaled plaque which appears on the skin in this disorder is the result of a vast acceleration of the usual skin replacement process or sloughing off, of the skin. A normal skin cell matures in twenty-one to forty days as it rises from the inner living layer of the epidermis to the outer surface of the keratin layer where it is shed from the body. At this external layer there is a constant invisible shedding of dead cells. In psoriasis it is believed that the cells transform themselves in two to seven days, and in such irregular manner that both the nucleated or parakeratotic living cells reach the skin surface together with the non-nucleated, or keratin, dead cells, forming together the psoriatic plaque. Since the nucleated cells are viable, they cannot shed themselves naturally therefore the presence of the plaque is the visible evidence of an incomplete sloughing of the skin. In the case of the reptile it would mean that it could not free itself wholly from the old skin, which would preclude its being discarded. In the human subject the vast acceleration which occurs, appears to be an increased dynamic effort on the part of the body to rid the individual of the outworn skin, replacing it rapidly with the new. However in so doing the harmony of the normal process of cell birth and death is disrupted. The human psoriatic lesion, therefore represents an intermediate form of keratinisation, between the reptilian level and the mammalian, and is the result of a special parakeratotic nucleated cell.

The bodily skin sites in a human subject which are prone in the normal course of events to repeated traumata are the elbow and the knees. Although these sites are the most commonly affected, any part of the body may be subject to this abnormal process.

The physical cause of the disorder has not yet been established medically. It appears to be initiated, in some instances, by shock or injury, in others by throat infections, and stress. Despite great advancements in dermatological therapeutic studies during recent years, psoriasis still remains a very difficult disorder to treat, and so far no cure has been established in the therapeutic field.

The above discourse reflects the inability of the psoriatic subject to cast his skin. There is immense mana attached to this natural process amongst primitive peoples who believe that by virtue of casting their skins certain animals, but in particular the serpent, renew their youth, and thus they never die. Such animals are believed to be immortal. There are countless myths based upon this theme whereby such creatures acquired eternal life, whereas man missed it and so had to die.

SYMBOLISM OF THE CAST SKIN

One such myth issues from Melanesia,[2] although it has a world-wide distribution. It illustrates how death came into the world.

> The good and malicious deities were conferring together concerning man after he had been made. The good deity remarked that mens' skin had begun to wrinkle. He continued to speak of their appearance, and added that although they were still young, they would become very ugly when they were old. He decided that when that happened, he would flay them, like an eel, and a new skin would grow, and thus men would renew their youth, like the snakes, and so become immortal. But the evil deity said "No it shall not be that way. When a man is old and ugly, we will dig a hole in the ground and put the body in it, and thus it shall always be among his descendants." Because the one who has the last word prevails, death came into the world.

A supportive myth from the Dusun tribe of Northern Borneo[3] reveals that man lost his immortality by error. When the creator god Kenharingan had made every living being he said "Who is able to cast his skin? If anyone can do so, he shall not die". The snake alone replied and said "I can". For this reason the snake does not die, unless killed by man. The Dusun tribe did not hear their creator god's question, or they would have thrown off their skin, and death would not have come into being. Already man had stopped listening to the voice of the creator.

To the primitive, and even today in the primitive in modern man, the extraordinary phenomenon of a serpent casting off its old dead skin, to emerge with some effort, glistening, supple, and alive with an apparently renewed youth is both fascinating and mysterious. Immortality by casting the skin is therefore a widespread conception, symbolic of transformation, and associated with a multiplicity of conjectures concerning death and rebirth.

A beautiful myth from Banks Island,[4] in the New Hebrides has a central theme which is found in countless others. Apparently at first men never died, they cast off their skins like snakes, and emerged with renewed youth. An old woman who was growing old went off to a stream to change her skin. According to some authorities she was the mother of the legendary hero Qat, to others she was Ul-ta-marama 'Change-skin of the world'. She threw off her old skin into the stream, and as it floated away she saw it catch upon a stick. She went home but her child refused to recognise her because he knew that his mother was an old woman, and not like the young woman who stood before him. So to pacify her child she went back to the river to retrieve the cast skin. Putting it on she returned again as an old woman to her child. From henceforward mankind ceased to cast the skin and men have died. In this group of myths too numerous to recount the old woman, or the old grandmother in some instances, signifies the unconscious where the transformation is initiated in the first place and carried through.

The psychological meaning attached to these myths is profound, touching upon the central essence of man's humanness. It indicates the development of an ability to discriminate between the opposites. The former state of pre-conscious wholeness of archaic man, where all opposites co-existed was sundered by the emerging presence of new ideas. Particularly so in the case of these myths concerning old age with its apparent uselessness and death as the opposite counterpoints of youth with its abundant promise in the fullness of life.

In the collective psyche the energic transformation responsible for the living reality of these universal myths produced the shedding of outdated attitudes, in order to permit the institution of the new. With the psychological awareness of the opposites brought by this increase of perception, slowly over thousands of years man has come to consciousness of his own being, a transformation process without end. Such myths are still active in man's psyche, as is evident in every life, fortunate enough to reach the middle years of existence. For it is then that psychic recognition of man's mortality and the absoluteness of death, confronts ego consciousness of the individual. The continued development of psychic life is essential for without the shedding of old attitudes, outmoded ideas, and outdated adaptations stagnation results and even death may occur. Skin casting is symbolic of soul change or psychic adaptation.

As has been observed, in those individuals who develop psoriasis the affected skin contains both living and dead cells impeded in the natural process of shedding by a non-differentiation. The conclusion cannot be avoided that their situation is exactly that of a serpent caught in the struggle to escape from its old and dead integument, which has become constricting. Should it fail to do so, it may die. It has to free itself in order to live. So it is with the human being whose psoriatic skin is the reflection of an à priori defective psychic adaptation. The flow of libido has suffered an obstruction by a content, a complex or an archetype, and stagnation or regression has occurred. Psychologically perhaps, it appears superficially, that an important step has been avoided, because of hesitation, laziness, fear or simply of unawareness of the necessity for change. On a deeper level the inner unconscious world reflects morbidity, in that certain aspects of life have remained unlived, be it in the intellectual, emotional, spiritual or sexual spheres, thus accounting for death in life.

The following cases in some small measure illustrate the psychic situation of the individual which has led to the development of the disorder. In each, the dermatosis is the gateway to a further step in the individuation process of the human being. Many years before I was introduced to Jung's psychology, I treated a middle aged man who suffered from psoriasis. Of all the thousands of patients I have seen as a physician he is the most unforgettable. It was through my encounter with this man that the psyche revealed to me, its impressive power.

I had just taken up my duties as a specialist and the encounter occurred during the first week, in which incidentally I had been inundated by a large number of new skin patients. This situation is not uncommon since those sufferers with long standing skin ailments are always eager to seek new advice. The majority of chronic skin diseases are resistant to treatment.

At the end of a long and tiring day the last patient was ushered into the consulting room. The man, himself had waited patiently to see me. He was fifty-eight years old, quietly spoken, and of an agreeable countenance. He told me he had suffered from severe psoriasis for many years. He had visited countless doctors throughout his life, without success. I examined him, and found that his entire body surface, including the scalp and face was affected with psoriasis. The whole body skin was covered with silvery scales, and was of a bright red colour. Since the disorder is common and treatment not conclusive, most dermatologists naturally feel a great despondency when they are presented with such severe cases. It is now over a quarter of a century since this event took place, but the therapy for the condition has not advanced in any great respect, since that time.

The patient told me that the dermatosis had started at the age of eighteen years, and he had never been free of it since. During the subsequent forty years he had always had an overtly psoriatic skin.

A silence descended between us, and I felt very weary. Suddenly he asked me "Do you think I will ever get better doctor?" For some singularly curious reason, quite inexplicable to me at that time, and totally out of character I said to him "You are in the wrong skin, in the wrong time, and in the wrong place". As the words tumbled out, I was immediately shocked, the patient needless to say, was stunned. He looked at me, and wordlessly nodded his head. In the ensuing silence, we stared at each other. He then got up slowly and departed. I do not know whether he said anything but I cannot recall that he did. I felt as I uttered the words, a strange instant feeling of exhilaration, which was only of a moment's duration, for it was followed at once, by an overwhelming sense of perplexity. I could not think why I had said such a thing. My discomfiture was intermingled with a sense of shame at my unpardonable lapse, but it did not obliterate the bewilderment at the bizarre nature of the statement itself. Furthermore I knew I had shocked the man to the essence of his being, since it is not customary for doctors to be quite so unsympathetic.

One week later, he returned to the clinic, without an appointment. He came on the off-chance that he might avail himself of a cancellation. When the clinic sister advised me of his presence I had him admitted at once. He entered, holding out his hands for me to see. There was not a blemish on the skin. The red and scaly plaques had disappeared, the finger nails which had all been involved with psoriasis on the previous visit remained as they were. His scalp and face were normal, and later when I examined his body, I found that the skin had reverted to normal. I was utterly astounded, so much that I wondered if it was the same man. We sat down together and he told me the following story.

After meeting me, he decided that he would walk home slowly so that he could think about that which I had said to him. During his solitary excursion he had come to realize that the statement I had made was exactly the truth in his case. When he arrived home he related the story to his wife, and explained all that had transpired. His wife made several derogatory remarks about my approach to the problem, but the patient reaffirmed to her that I was correct. The next day after this revelation (for indeed it was) he changed his entire life.

The patient was a master butcher and was both the son, grandson, and great-grandson of master butchers. At the age of eighteen years he was apprenticed to his father, and so began the learning process as he unquestioningly followed his ancestral footsteps. He was very successful, and succeeded in building up an excellent business, which eventually included several shops. However, as he explained, at eighteen he did not want to be a butcher, he did not like the trade, and had never liked it. The part which he rebelled against, most particularly was the slaughter of the young animals. He said in describing this "It goes against the grain". The day after his realization he said to his wife 'By God that doctor is right'. He decided at once to sell his shops, and within twenty-four hours, they were on the market. In the subsequent twenty-four hours he began his search for a farm. In explanation he added, 'Now I shall rear animals, instead of killing them'. He also stated that from the moment he realized he was working against his inner nature his skin began to get better, and within a week, on the occasion, of his next hospital visit, the psoriasis had cleared.

Undoubtedly my completely spontaneous comment upon his situation had come directly from the unconscious, and at that time I had no conscious understanding of its meaning. The fact that it triggered off an instantaneous healing process, proved the wisdom of the unconscious in this man's case. It is perfectly understandable to me today, in the wisdom of years of analytical training, but at that time, the statement and its incredible effect disturbed me profoundly. Since I had not intended to make such a remark, fortunately the ego did not seek to grasp any self-adulation. The patient and I regarded it as a miracle, which it was. The statement itself had proved to be particularly apt, "in the wrong skin, in the wrong time, and in the wrong place".

As we have seen, the patient's situation was similar to that of a serpent which has not the strength to shed its old skin. The emerging sleek and handsome reptile with its new and glistening skin has become a symbol for longevity, immortality, and rebirth.

The image of the patient as a serpent unable to cast its skin is singularly precise, histiologically speaking. The skin as the garment of the body signifies an attitude or adaptation, which requires to be changed, shed or cast off as it were, since its presence is no longer conducive for the subject's well-being.

The butcher had married, like his father and grandfather before him, he had raised a family, and made a successful adaptation to the material side of life. He was however always dissatisfied he did not like the work, particularly the killing, it went 'against the grain'. His anima reacted negatively towards this aspect of his life, and undoubtedly had always done so. She it was who was instrumental in his seeking new advice, for on the occasion of his first visit he, explained that he wished to see me because, I was a woman specialist. He had thought a woman might have a different approach. His visit therefore was a propitiation for the anima, and was the first step to his recovery.

The anima as the archetype of life and also of fate seeks to involve a man in life. Slowly over the years, a silent transformation had been taking place in the unconscious and so it came about that at last he was able to listen to the inner feminine and to heed her voice. In reality he had had an intuitive feeling that he should once again seek help. The inner transformation resulted in a new attitude which paved the way to the subsequent outer rebirth. He had become receptive, and his reflections after the fateful meeting substantiates this fact. It is clear from this man's long history of suffering, a period of forty years, represented symbolically the impediment which existed between ego consciousness and the unconscious psyche. Here was an individual who had suppressed his instinctual reactions and had thereby cut himself off from the unconscious.

Over many decades the observation of countless psoriatic sufferers has led me to the view that in spite of outer appearances there is almost always an innate sloth, or covert indolence concealed in the character of many of the victims. Usually the visible character reveals a high energy potential, motivated and excessively occupied and with a steady perseverance to achieve and maintain self-imposed high standards of perfection. Often an apparently relaxed attitude to the disorder belies an underlying desperate need for a cure, which is counteracted by an equally desperate effort to avoid it. Insight into the condition is common, and the adverse effects of stress and anxiety are well known and recognised by the subject. However there is a tendency to hide the body, partly because of adverse comment but chiefly because of a sense of uncleanness, which leads eventually to a psychological suppression of the body. In many psoriatic subjects the body as the despised shadow is neglected, frequently abused and sometimes totally ignored. In such individuals there is a strong inclination to allow the psoriasis to become florid and extensive, through neglect.

THE INDOLENT MAN.

Such a psoriatic subject visited me in order to enquire what medicaments were available to clear the condition. This man had a particularly fine intellect, he was married, had a devoted wife and a family of daughters. The skin disorder had plagued him for most of his married life, a period of several years. I spent a long time explaining how with care he could undoubtedly clear the lesions, and with the assiduous application of unguenta involving about a quarter of an hour per day, maintain the skin in apparent normality. He paid the strictest attention to my discourse, took notes, and departed in high spirits. His next appearance, due a few weeks later was cancelled, and in its place I received a charming note, in which he explained that he had not undertaken the therapy, he found it too laborious to apply the creams and lotions, and the regimen I had suggested was too tedious. He added, by way of a postscript, "I am glad to know that should the need arise the condition can be cleared". As I read it I did wonder just what the need could be to which he referred. Severe psoriasis where most of the body skin is afflicted produces a daily shedding of skin, which litters the bed upon which the subject sleeps, and the bedroom floor as the friction of the clothing causes the scaly plaques to be rubbed off and dislodged from the skin in the course of the night. Such indolence as described, on the part of this man with regard to the personal care of his body, is encompassed in the deadly sin of sloth. He was unconscious of his shadow and had little conception of the effect he had upon his family, the members of which undoubtedly carried his feeling function to a very great extent.

He was a man of unquestioned talent and had an obvious gift for a witty turn of phrase, combined with a cynical eye for human existence. However behind this agreeable persona, there was a sense of chilling isolation. Apparently he had been the idolized only son of a devoted and indulgent mother, whose death allowed him to find a wife of the same ilk. Fate decreed that he was to sire only daughters, so in this enclosed feminine world he had never 'felt the need' to take up the problem of his anima. As the archetype of life she would undoubtedly force him out of the prison of the mother complex in which he had remained inert, unmoving and lulled like a child for over five decades of his life. He could not bring himself to change his attitude, he remained firmly ensconced in the neurosis, only his skin exhibited a reaction to the unconscious indolence, of his personality. He could not symbolically shed his skin, and achieve a higher conscious level, and therefore became afraid when the chance to do so presented itself.

THE TRAVELLING SALESMAN

A much younger man presented himself for therapy with an equally severe psoriasis. He exhibited indolence in a completely different way. Outwardly there was a singular air of desperation, with an intensity which was unnerving. He had visited several of the most prestigious centres of dermatological excellence in his endeavour to find a cure. Alas he had no success, so he began to study the condition, much as would a medical student. He became completely involved and highly knowledgeable concerning all the physical facts of the disorder.

At the time he presented himself to me for psychological advice he was thirty-two years old. The psoriatic disorder had appeared suddenly about five years earlier, at the time of his mother's death. He was occupied as the sales consultant-in-chief for the family business, but lived at home, with his parents. After his mother's death, his father introduced his mistress of many years into the family home, and the young man was told to leave at once. This he did, without demur, and found that he had no dwelling place. So he lost his mother, his home, and his roots all at the same time. It was exactly then that the psoriasis had started. He had an excellent grasp of the intricacies of the family business and because of his expertise, his occupation came to involve constant world-wide travelling, at the behest of his father. His uprootedness was enhanced further by this development. Although he bought a house for himself he rarely had the time to visit it. He was not able to continue his former friendships or establish close ties with his peers of either sex. He was in fact a very lonely man. The most disturbing fact of his life was that of the telephone call. Every second night his father telephoned him to enquire about the business, no matter in what part of the world he happened to be. When he arrived home, the first thing he did was to let his father know that he had returned with the sales figures.

In the subsequent analysis it became clear to him that his father was a ruthless tyrant, who treated his son as a slave. It was very difficult for him to accept this fact, as he held his father in high esteem, and projected his own well developed feeling upon the parent. It required many months and considerable courage on his part before he could stand up to his father's domination. Eventually he came to understand the father complex, and began to realize that he treated his own body exactly as his father treated him. He rejected it, misused it and did not permit it to be 'earthed'. At long last he managed to establish a semi-permanent home abroad, and found a congenial lady companion. This was the beginning of the liberation.

This young man had a curious distraught appearance at the beginning of the analysis, and I had the impression that he resembled nothing so much as a wounded animal which indeed he was. He reached a point where he understood the psychic dynamics of the situation as well as he had understood the psoriatic disorder, but he could not muster up the courage to break with his father. He had been closely bound to the mother, and had not the sufficient ruthlessness to stand firm against the tyrant. Each time a crisis approached, he was well prepared, but at the last moment, he could not 'cast the skin' and each time returned to his former situation. It was noteworthy that every psychic lapse, brought an exacerbation of the psoriasis.

THE FINANCIER

Another clear example of a psoriatic subject caught in an insoluble situation was a man of about fifty years of age, who presented himself for psychotherapy in the early nineteen seventies. He had developed psoriasis when he was a young man and had suffered from an extensive and severe form of the disorder during the subsequent thirty years. He had been hospitalized on several occasions and had received steroid therapy over a prolonged period. This was followed by a long period of ill health due to the side effects of the steroids. His metier was that of a financial consultant, and he worked for a major corporation. When he was about fifty, his firm moved him to another region. His displacement was only the second time he had left the city of his birth, the first was during the war when he was a soldier.

At the onset of psychotherapy he was in fact seriously ill. In the previous dermatological centre, he had been given a cytotoxic drug after the steroid therapy, and he had suffered hepatotoxicity. It was therefore essential to treat his skin disorder conservatively. The analysis revealed a curious event. During the war whilst serving abroad with the Armed Forces the psoriasis cleared up completely. He said that in Africa it was very hot, and he, like his colleagues removed his shirt. He said "for the first time in my life I felt warm". The sun, he thought had cleared the disorder.

It transpired that his psoriasis had actually started the month following his first meeting with his future wife-to-be. He married her before the war, so the war also produced a long separation from his spouse. Prior to his marriage he had begun to train in the world of accounting at the express wish of his parents, particularly his mother who thought he should have a safe job. His fiancée supported his mother. He had wanted to serve in the Armed Forces, when he left school, but was not permitted. He got his chance however, when the war provided the opportunity. In explaining about the Army service he said that he had never been happier. On his return home after the war, he returned to his old job, and quickly ascended the ladder of promotion, eventually to reach the top of his profession. His marriage apparently prospered, his wife, was described by him in glowing terms, and he could not be blessed with better children. As I listened to such a remarkable account of domestic bliss I wondered why he had been stricken with psoriasis.

The analysis revealed the inner story. It became clear that the anima as fate had served him a hard blow in leading him to the particular lady he was to marry. It came to light through his dreams that she was a woman of iron will which was disguised under an apparent sweet and gentle nature. As the dreams pounded him with an onslaught of images revealing her true nature, he could not bring himself to see it, or comprehend it. During the analysis he was hospitalized three times, for acute exacerbation of his psoriatic disorder. Each time he basked in the care and attention provided by the nursing staff, his psoriasis cleared away and he always emerged sleek, and handsome exactly as would a snake, after it has shed its skin. Within a month of his return to his home on each occasion, the psoriasis returned.

It was made very clear that the unconscious nature of his wife was not conducive for his well being. It was further pointed out that he also had a cold blooded inner nature, which disabused him, and treated him with disrespect, exactly as did his wife. But sadly he could not bring himself to believe it, there was a sullen and deep resistance to this truth. So the psoriasis remained. I realized after about five years that perhaps in this deeply unconscious marriage he was in some way protected, and it was his fate to remain a severely affected psoriatic subject. The dissociation between the conscious and the unconscious was not to be bridged at that time.

THE DOCTOR

A parallel case history concerned a physician, a particularly scholarly man who had suffered from a mild form of the disorder since his marriage. Outwardly he had the appearance of a kindly patriarchal figure, which was accentuated by his deep interest and involvement in spiritual and ecclesiastical matters. He was a constant and regular church attender presiding over several church committees and spoke frequently and eloquently about the state of his soul. Church music was his passion and his greatest pleasure was to ensconce himself in a dark corner of some mediæval church, and allow himself to be wafted away by organ music. His days were spent working as a physician, his evenings serving on countless committees or listening to church music and the weekends were entirely devoted to either scholarly activities or matters of the church. He spoke rarely of his wife, but when he did there was a curious reverential tone as if he was speaking of a divine presence. He spoke even more rarely of his grown-up children.

Here was an introverted man whose major function was thinking, and with a well developed practical side he was adept with bureaucratic council and committee matters. He had never developed his feeling side, indeed he was unaware of it, but like so many possessed of an unkind, or indeed cold heart, he was overly sentimental. Undoubtedly his intellect was exceptional but the accompanying semblance of benignity was usually dispersed with alacrity, for he had a subtly barbed tongue, serpentine in its darting wounding quality. He had the ability and the malicious wit, to injure by a well chosen word or a cleverly turned phrase. He made enemies easily by these means, and alienated himself from those who would be his friends. His rhetorical skills employed remarks in such manner that they flew to the heart of the victim as a precisely aimed knife is able to pierce the flesh. The unexpected nature of the attack and particularly its speed was witch-like. The witch is one who furthers the bad, and moreover her attack is always given without preparation or warning. That is the secret of its devastating nature, indeed here was the problem. Undeniably he was an excellent doctor, and certainly he did present a benign persona, which was alas all too easily transformed into what can only be described as a spitting cat. His anima was a spiteful and malevolent being, and since possessed by her, he had no control when she decided to sting pierce or wound another. Thus he became an unloved and solitary man, he was uninvolved in life and wrapped as it were in layers of scholarly winding sheets. The rapid turnover of the epidermal cells, and the inability to cast off the nucleated psoriatic cells, revealed his general life situation. His frantic activities when every moment was occupied concealed the inner total inertia where nothing ever changed, and the status quo was maintained. The psoriasis was the body's intense effort urging for an increase of conscious awareness.

He was possessed of two unusual characteristics. One was a frightening antipathy to all things of a psychological nature, he would exhibit insensate rage if one of his peers should put forward a theorem recognising a possible psychic cause to somatic illness. His intense concern regarding the soul did not correlate with the fact that the soul as an inner feminine being is within the province of man himself. He spoke of the soul as an unapproachable pure, unsullied, divine being, in heaven. This attitude revealed a deep split in his feminine unconscious, and accounted for the total negativity which was on occasion directed against any woman who happened to be in his vicinity, be they old, infirm, or young and healthy. The second characteristic was a habit. From time to time and without apparent cause,

103

he would begin to twirl the gold wedding ring which he wore on the right hand. Sometimes it whirled so rapidly that it would spin off and sail across the room. There never seemed to be a reason why this act should intervene in a conversation. Without doubt, the marital situation was problematical, but since such a man would never contemplate analysis, any thoughts must perforce remain conjectural.

On one occasion he mentioned that as a young man, he had passed several months in a European city where he had had the most wonderful time of his life. By a strange coincidence, which later proved to be a synchronistic event, some years ago I found myself on a transatlantic flight. I was seated next to an elderly European woman who in the course of conversation revealed that as a young woman she had known this man. She spoke of him warmly and it transpired that she had been a great friend of his in those far off days of their youth. She it was who had been the companion who had made those hours, so idyllic. Some months later I was to learn quite by chance, that the man had died, and as I discovered in due course, the death had occurred about the time his old friend and I were speaking of him.

The anima problem was of the greatest importance in this life, the marriage was most probably a social marriage, and his wife was for him in consciousness an unsullied goddess. The psoriasis was the marker of the fact that he was caught in a trap and could not escape, because he was not prepared to admit that he himself was mistaken, therefore not perfect, and also that his lady-wife likewise left a great deal to be desired. The inability to change his attitude is symbolized by the serpent's incapacity to change its skin. His serpentine venomous attacks upon women was the price he paid for his unconsciousness. As soon as he retired from practice he became ill and died within a few weeks. The prospect of living with the outer goddess and the inner witch was too daunting for him, and in death he found the escape.

One cannot but surmise what the outcome would have been if he had pursued the love of his youth. Undoubtedly the parting at that time represented a fateful step, in his life.

THE MEN WHO ESCAPED THE HOLOCAUST

It might be interesting to relate an unusual incident which occurred some years after the Second World War. At the time I was working at a medical school teaching hospital dermatological clinic and during this period it was my privilege to meet round about the same time, two unrelated elderly Jewish men, who had been in the same concentration camp in Germany during the war. They had each escaped the gas chamber by great good fortune, although they were not known to each other. Each presented himself separately at my clinic within a matter of weeks.

They were both well advanced in years and extremely obese. One was a

Jew from the Netherlands, and the other from a Central European country.

As has been exceedingly well documented the German Camp Commandants and their assistant staff sought out all those patients who were maimed, crippled, disfigured or suffered a serious illness. The purpose was to arrange execution in the gas chambers as expediently as possible. As can be imagined, the numbers for the execution chambers were vast, and since food supplies, towards the end of the war were depleted, it was decided to limit food intake for those waiting execution. One meal of black bread and a cup of soup were provided over a twenty-four hour period. The waiting list for death was about eight weeks, consequently all the intended victims lost a great deal of weight on this starvation diet. Although the details varied slightly the two men were quite adamant on the following points. As soon as the inmates reached the point where death was imminent, they were re-examined by the camp doctors, and all those who remained in a parlous state went forward to their deaths. However Germanic meticulousness did not permit execution if for any odd chance, the physical deformity or malady had cleared up, and so these fortunates were spared.

The two patients were grossly overweight, and both had suffered from intractable psoriasis for most of their lives. In each case, in the eight weeks or so of waiting, they lost weight, several stones, and in the case of these two particular patients, the psoriasis disappeared. Consequently, when examined again finally, since they were healthy, and the skin was clear, they were released from the sentence of death. Later when the camps were cleared needless to say they were some of the few who survived. Each man, individually told me that a number of people suffering from psoriasis all recovered and by this happening, all their lives were saved.

Psoriasis does undergo spontaneous resolution from time to time, of this there is no doubt, but it appears incongruous, that at such a time, it should disappear.

Their attendance at the clinic was for therapy for the psoriasis which had recurred. Both men were as stated once again obese, and both exhibited severe generalised psoriasis.

The rational explanation was that the rapid loss of weight with lowered cholesterol levels had somehow been instrumental in the clearance. The fact that the subsequent weight gain was accompanied by a recrudescence of the disorder appeared to substantiate the hypothesis. This however hardly satisfies an analytical turn of mind. Since a psychological approach had not been previously attempted or considered, neither of the old men was in a position to explain the feelings and emotions at the time of their impending death, and subsequent reprieve, which was already about twenty years in the past. Admittedly although each spoke the English tongue, their grasp of the language was limited, but by means of interpreters I was able to discover a few salient facts.

Both men had been successful businessmen in their respective countries, and although members of their families had disappeared the immediate family in each case had survived. This enabled each to re-commence life with more or less intact family units. A curious fact which emerged was that neither of the men regarded their escape as miraculous. Both of them were completely unconscious of the divine grace which had been afforded to them, and appeared to have felt no gratitude at the merciful escape which had presented itself to them, by way of their mutual skin disease. The fact that in each case, it cleared spontaneously, would betoken that each had developed a different approach or attitude to life. Since death seemed to be irrevocable, and life was no longer the problem, the change of attitude was most probably associated with this fact. One of the men had lived all his life in a ghetto, and the other in a tightly-knit Jewish community. It is not unreasonable to assume that having lived their lives collectively, sudden death had to be faced in an individual way, albeit thousands were facing death together. It would seem that when the death sentence was pronounced each of the two men accepted it as an individual reality, and by so doing the skin reflected the inner equilibrium.

The fact that they both regained weight and their psoriasis after the war, indicates that neither had been conscious of the new awareness of individuality, the reality of which slowly sank away back into oblivion, when the danger was passed and the collective nature of their lives once again assumed control. In each case perhaps a vital step in the individuation process was not taken.

When the python which is reputed to be a good mother, completes its egg laying, it curls its body round the eggs and remains in this position for two months. During this period of incubation, until the eggs are hatched this cold blooded creature, whose temperature is normally close to that of its environment, becomes feverish and suffers intense thirst, and lack of appetite. The temperature in the coils of its body sometimes rises as much as fifteen degrees. It appears that in the reptile there is an archaic type of emotional reaction sufficient to cause a rise in temperature and accompanying signs of nervousness. The emotionality, if use of this term can be permitted, belongs to the deepest instinctual strata of existence where primitive maternal emotionalism is vitally concerned with the life process, and death is the greatest enemy.

Perhaps the approach of death with its terrors posed sufficient threat to touch a deeply unconscious archaical or primitive emotionality in each of these men, which was of sufficient strength to overcome the dissociation between ego consciousness, and the inner emotional world. Albeit, the healing although only momentarily present, it was enough to initiate changes at the primitive epidermal cell level and permit a normal developmental shedding of the parakeratotic cell. It signifies nothing less than a transformation from a reptilian stage of development to a human one.

Psychologically, neither of these men had contact with their individual inner emotional world.

REFERENCES

1 Spearman, R. I. C., Biological Reviews, Vol. 41., p. 59, February 1966.
2 Mythology of All Races, Vol. IX, p. 118.
3 Ibid., p. 182.
4 Frazer, J. G., Folk Lore in the Old Testament, p. 28, Macmillan & Co. Ltd., London 1923.

7

LICHEN PLANUS
(Lichen Rubra Planus)

Lichen planus is a skin disease which is characterized by flat smooth bluish-red plaques on the skin, ranging from the tiniest single papule to agglomerations of considerable size, covering large surface areas of the body skin.

The appearance of the condition in the past was apparently suggestive of an alien parasitic growth which lodged itself on the skin and slowly encroached upon the healthy areas. Consequently and pertinently the descriptive name of lichen plans (flat lichen) was given to it. Lichens are the tiny unicellular organisms, which cling tenaciously and apparently without sustenance to the windward side of the weathered stone on the walls of churches, old buildings and tombstones, as well as the bark of trees, producing a superimposed brilliant green patina over the underlying surface. The dermatosis is not due to an infection, fungal or otherwise, and its ætiology is as yet unknown.

The unique lesion which is central to the disease is a flat topped papule of a peculiar violaceous colour often described as livid. It is possessed of a pearly opalescent sheen, when viewed obliquely and its shape is polyhedral. This papule itself is diagnostic of the disease. The symptom which brings the patient for therapy apart from the presence of the eruption itself, is irritation. Lichen planus like many other dermatoses mentioned, can produce its own 'furor dermaticus'. The striking feature however is the lividity of the papule resembling exactly the skin change appearing on the cadaver a few hours after death.

Since the physical cause has yet to be identified, the treatment remains problematical, and is therefore symptomatic. Steroid therapy is often essential and of great value in severe cases with mouth scalp and genital involvement. In such instances, subsequent damage may be mutilating without recourse to the more potent medicaments.

THE WOMAN WITH THE FATHER COMPLEX

A charming woman in her early forties was referred by her private practitioner for dermatological diagnosis because over a period of several months, she had developed what he thought was a devastating creeping eruption due to a fungal infection which covered her entire body, and had involved the mucous membrane of her mouth. Fortunately the scalp and genital areas were uninvolved.

She was intensely afraid, and had become both distressed and fatigued with the severe irritation. The fear is easily understood. The appearance of Lichen planus is unusual, it has about it a still, and deathly quality. It also has the look of permanence, and one often wonders just how such an apparently solid change in the skin will ever again transform itself into the normality of healthy tissue. Such is the transforming power of the skin however that even large plaques over periods of months and sometimes years do eventually revert to the former condition, although scarring is often a possibility.

Apart from the psychic distress occasioned by the disease itself, she admitted to no other fear or anxiety. She stressed that her marriage of many years was satisfactory, she had no complaints about her children, or her family. Everything it seemed was in a state of harmony except, her skin which plagued her to distraction, and had the appearance of a cadaver.

With steroid therapy, nursing care and rest, she began to improve slowly at first, and then more rapidly when her confidence improved, and a rapport was established with her attendants. It was explained to her that Lichen planus is often difficult to resolve completely and sometimes is long lasting and the inadvisability of prolonged steroid therapy would have to be considered, because of serious side effects. In view of these facts a suggestion was proffered that she might like to air anything of a problematical nature existing in her life. After a period of several weeks she admitted that for some years she had been beset by a terrible fear. She had married twenty years earlier, and her marriage was very happy, she was the mother of two children of whom she was very fond but they came second to her husband to whom she was devoted.

Prior to the onset of the skin disorder she had developed a phobia. She had become possessed by a fear that her husband was going to die. This always occurred during the night time. She added that she could not live without him, for 'he was her life'. When she described the fear, she became quite pale, and did in fact lose her voice as she relived the terror. She had never previously discussed this problem, with her husband or another. Over a period of weeks, as the fear attached to this aspect of her life became less acute, another problem moved into focus, it was that of the father complex. The father was undoubtedly the dominant parent, whilst the mother played a shadowy background rôle. Indeed she was so insubstantial, that at first it seemed that she had died, she was so rarely spoken of. The sis-

109

ters of the woman had left home to be married before they were twenty years old, and she described their marriages as less than ideal, when compared to her own.

The father was a clergyman in his late fifties, apparently energetic handsome extremely popular with his parishioners, especially the women. He was it seemed outwardly fond of his wife, but did not permit her to make any major decisions regarding the household or the children. She was solely a house-wife, and his companion in parochial duties only. Early in the analysis, the woman described a dream in which she was lying in her own bed, as a young girl, and her father was standing at the foot of her bed staring at her. In describing the dream, she was able to relate that the emotion which she felt on waking was the same terror which she experienced when she was gripped by the fear of her husband's death. This image proved to be the turning point in her analysis. Prior to the dream she had always protected her father, and made excuses for him, but after the dream she was able to face the fact that her father was an unmitigated tyrant.

It came to light that during the years of her girlhood, she and her sisters were made to attend one hour of bible reading each evening before supper. No matter how hungry the children were or whether or not the father was late, the reading took place every day. Later as they grew older and approached womanhood, it became his habit to question every aspect of their lives, and nightly he adjured them not to sleep with men until they married. As their marriages approached he made each swear on the bible that she had not lost her virginity.

After the woman herself had married it became customary for the father to telephone her at least every week, and as the years passed these telephone calls became more frequent. If she happened to be out when he called, she was expected to telephone on her return, if not she was always chastised. At the time of her illness the father had taken to telephoning her daily. He never spoke against her husband but he intimated that she was not being cared for as he always cared for their mother.

The father, a paragon of virtue believed that the sanctity of marriage should be preserved and moreover the husband as head of the household was responsible for its maintenance. This kindly solicitous paternal clerk in holy orders, had however another side to his character. He had always had, and still possessed a propensity for illicit sexual affairs amongst the women of his parish. His wife and daughters suffered the gossip and the anxiety, but each was so afraid of his tyranny and his outbursts of rage, that they could not confront him with the fact of his less than perfect side, his shadow.

Much later when she was beginning to get better, she was asked again about the feeling of terror which she had experienced upon waking from the dream of her father. She then admitted as a child, and as a young girl, she had prayed every night for her father to die. Moreover, as a young woman, she had often wished him dead. The prayer and the secret wish had

110

fallen away, as she had grown up, married, and left home. Just prior to the onset of the lichen planus, she had learned from her mother that her father had had a particularly unsavoury escapade with a woman who had threatened to blackmail him. The family had joined forces to support both parents, but the woman said that she no longer felt the inclination to do so. She was of the view that the recent bombardment from her father by means of the telephone was to ensure that she would stand by him through his difficulties. Just as the skin disease made itself apparent, the father escaped from public condemnation by a hair's breadth, and immediately resumed the mantle of his former arrogance. Then it was that the eruption appeared.

The case demonstrates how an unconscious father complex can dominate and disrupt a life. Her childhood and girlhood had been overshadowed by the dissociation in the personality of the father. The apparent escape into marriage did not save her from a brutal tormenting animus. It is the father who provides the first masculine image for his daughter. In this case it is clear she had suffered untold distress at the hands of the brutal and sadistic shadow of this deeply unconscious man. Her father did not practice that which he preached, on the one hand he advocated the sanctity of marriage whilst on the other he destroyed it. As head of the household, his concern for his wife's feelings was hardly evident, throughout the years.

The patient however possessed an inner sadistic animus, by supporting her father, she suppressed her true feelings allowing her father to dominate her, she did not give credence to her own feminine personality. By accepting her father's double standards she became at odds with herself. She was able to live in apparent contentment, but underneath was a serious unconscious disturbance. She had wished her father dead, indeed prayed for it, those wishes although long ago fallen into the unconscious were alive, and vibrant since possessed of a dynamism of their own. She was punished for the wickedness of her secret wish twenty years later, when in spite of her maturity she had not yet come to terms, with the truth of her father's character, where behind the pious persona lurked a devilish tormentor. Her animus secretly whispered to her in the dead of night, as she lay with her husband, 'What if he should die'? What indeed, for then she would again be face to face with the father.

The husband had as a positive animus figure, shielded her, and protected her against the inner tyrant for over two decades, almost half her life.

The most recent escapade of the father, was in fact for her the death of the false image. At last she had to face the truth of his character. Since however she was at that time unaware of her inner complex, she believed the brutal nightly thought was her own, and so she lived in terror. One sees here, a drama being enacted in the unconscious, which in consciousness is revealed by a disturbing night thought, and an irritating rash on the skin. The latter was the means by which she came to consciousness of her inner self. She was able to learn, of the outer dissociated father, her own sadistic inner masculine being, and her own weakness in the feminine sphere. The eruption signified the death of the father's power over her life, and a coming to terms with the inner figure. This woman, after a year and a half made a complete recovery without skin scarring. Moreover her psychic problem was brought to consciousness and the presence of the father problem realized in her life. In the following years she grew to understand her father, and in so doing was able to consolidate her own marriage.

In retrospect, the irritation of the lichen planus symbolized the deep irritation which occurred in her psyche. At the time of the eruption, there had already been a death, for she had at last faced the fact of her father's dissociation, and her false attitude towards him had died. In this case, undoubtedly the disease itself, was the portent of the healing of psyche which was to follow, in the course of time. Without psychotherapy, the changes would have most probably continued, but consciousness of the inner drama would have been absent. For this woman, lichen planus was an important step in her individuation process, coming to consciousness of self.

THE MAN WITH THE TWO CALVES

A man of forty-eight years of age, had noticed, six months previously a strange bluish rash which had begun to cover most of his body. He had sought help, but the general practitioner was not sure of the diagnosis. This is not uncommon, since the pattern of the disease itself has an unexpected quality, and a strange air of permanence, which combined with the lividity is puzzling to an untrained eye.

The man was a senior foreman in a large engineering shop. He had begun life as an apprentice, and worked his way up. It was a responsible job, and there had been a good deal of stress during the previous years, on account of the problems of labour, and associated political unrest. He had been working long hours, and he thought that the rash might be due to fatigue, and anxiety.

He was married and the father of three well grown children. His marriage was happy, and he and his wife got on together.

Some years previously he had bought a small holding in the country, a farm, with some land, in preparation for his retirement. He intended eventually to build it up into a working farm. In order to do this he had decided to work long overtime shifts at the engineering works. When he had completed the farm buildings, most of which he restored himself, he began to buy the required machinery and finally he was ready to buy the stock. His first purchase was that of twin calves. He decided as they were so small, to keep them in an outhouse at his home, and so each night as soon as he came home, he fed them and cared for them.

All through the winter, he looked after them and when they were seven months old, they caught an infection. He said that he noticed that one calf had developed running eyes, so he called a veterinary surgeon, who came at once. He pronounced that the little calf had a virus infection, and thought it was serious. The following day, it died; then the day afterwards, the second calf developed the same symptoms and twenty-four hours later it also died. All this had taken place, six months previously. It was only when he was asked about the onset of the bluish eruption on his body that he remembered these facts concerning his calves. As he remembered the details, he explained that he associated the appearance of the rash with the death of the calves. Suddenly as he recalled the details, and told the story, he started to sob. His whole body was wracked with the deepest of profound shudders. I have never experienced such extraordinary convulsions caused by emotion in a man before. I realized that the deepest strata of his being had been touched, in a most extraordinary way. The weeping lasted for several minutes, then it was over. He then straightened up, and said 'That's it, that's what caused the rash, I shall be better now'. He was quite correct. I saw him once more some weeks later, and he had recovered. He received no therapy for the illness.

It is many years since I saw him and I did not discover any other details of his life. He remains vividly in my memory because of the passion of his weeping, and I always wondered what lay behind such a profound reaction. I have seen many people weep in my life, but never have I witnessed such a storm before or since. Since there was no way of obtaining further knowledge of this man, other than that which he had given to me, the matter lapsed and I forgot the episode. However many years later, a book fell into my hands concerning love and culture crisis in Ancient Greece.[1] In it, I read of 'Koukoudi'. Apparently among the myriad nameless demons and genii in rural Greece there is a specific demon conceived in human form called 'Koukoudi'. Even today in modern times it is still feared. Rituals are designed to ward off the Koukoudi, one of which is to plough a magic circle around the town using twin calves, which are then slaughtered and buried when the circle is complete. The modernized reason given as to why calves were used, is that they were on good terms with Christianity, since they licked Christ at his birth. However smallpox, cholera and plague are personified in Greece and Europe as women, even today. In the Greek language koukoudi is a pimple, a bump, or a nodule, it is used for the lymph nodes in bubonic plague. On the other hand, the personalization of disease dates from ancient times for example the sphinx at Thebes was responsible for the pestilence there, and also Medusa herself was a pestilence bringer.

Koukoudi is similar to the pre-Germanic word kuzdo for kudtho, meaning hidden. The Latin cūdo means helmet, the Celtic word koudo means concealment. This can be compared to the Gothic Huzo and the Germanic Hozda both meaning hidden, which is related to the Middle and Old High German – Hort which means treasure and is similar to the English 'hoard'.

The motif of the twin calf sacrifice was to placate and ward off koukoudi, who brought illness in the shape of a skin disease. The personalization relates to the goddess and points to the archetypal image of the feminine in the unconscious.

What strange echoes were awakened in the psyche of this man to overwhelm him with such a storm of emotion? It is known that he had been employed for over thirty years in an engineering factory and had risen to be a senior foreman, and that he was both an industrious and a practical man. Moreover he had had the foresight to perceive the need for another occupation at his retirement, and to plan for it, by acquiring a small farm. He had then assiduously worked towards the goal. The essence of masculinity is to perceive the goal and work towards it. The acquisition of the first stock in the form of two calves, undoubtedly touched his feeling which was most probably his inferior function. The tending and caring for the young life was indubitably a new venture for him and one which pleased him enormously.

The sudden death of the little creatures in practical terms meant the not inconsiderable loss financially of his first stock, but does not explain the emotional storm, which followed, six months later. In all probability he had been cut off and separated from the world of nature, and the appropriation of the land was the first step to return to that world, and mitigate the separation. The calves would represent the future, and their care symbolized the maternalism required in any future farmer. Their unexpected death however reflected the irrational world of Nature, where in spite of care and attention accidents do happen and death does occur. The death also represented his sudden confrontation with this dark instinctual world of the feminine. To be overwhelmed by such an expression of deep sorrow meant that an archetype had been constellated in his psyche, flooding images and emotion into his being. Such weeping was for something mysterious and strange, and had about it a numinosum. Somewhere in his deep unconscious, his soul knew of ancient rituals, and the meaning of the divine sacrifice to the goddess. At the time of the death of the calves one suspects that no emotion was shown outwardly, and possibly he had only a fleeting feeling of sadness which did not reach consciousness and which quickly passed away afterwards. Then the rash of lichen planus presented itself, with the image of the death in the skin. The irritation inherent was to plague him until he sought therapy to ease himself. The simple question as to how the rash had started was the key to the immediate unlocking of the memory and the imprisoned emotion was released. The torrent racing through the opened flood gates, was the image conjured up, by the shuddering body, and the fall of tears.

One sees so often, the suffering occasioned by the Self in the process of individuation. In his case, the suffering would not have become conscious had not the rash or Koukoudi haunted him and urged him to seek aid, until such time as he realized its presence in his inner being. Then through the two minutes of deep emotion the long suppressed inner feeling was freed, and he was released. Psyche spoke severely to him, through the skin, because he had already unconsciously turned towards her realm.

THE MAN WITH THE PARALYSED SON

As stated, lichen planus can occur anywhere upon the body skin, and not uncommonly involves the scalp, mouth, and genitals. Sometimes a case may present with a single lesion only. In the following case history a man of forty-five years presented himself with lichen planus which had developed only on the male organ, but was of considerable severity, in that the urethral orifice was affected, by a partial obliteration.

The history which he gave was that the condition had appeared, two or three days after he had sustained a severe shock. Apparently whilst working in his garden he heard a screech of brakes, and witnessed his next-door neighbour whilst driving his motor car, accidentally run over a child. As he heard the impact he knew instinctively that it was his own son. The boy was nine years old and had been riding his bicycle. When the patient ran to see what had happened, he saw at once that it was his little son, and he thought that he had been killed. The boy however had not been, and did in fact survive the accident, but was to live the rest of his life as a quadraplegic. He had sustained a fracture of the cervical spine during the accident, with irreparable damage to the spinal cord just below the base of the skull.

At the time of the accident the neighbour who had driven the motor car was also in a state of shock and was very upset. However as soon as the question of court proceedings arose, on the advice of his lawyers he never again spoke to either the patient or his son. This was particularly sad, as the child had been very friendly with the neighbour before the accident. Within a few days after the tragedy, the skin eruption had appeared on the penis, but because of the shock and profound distress the patient did not notice it consciously for at least a week. Then he realized that something abnormal had occurred at the orifice of the penis. The explanation to him was that the condition was the result of the grave shock he had sustained, and this was undoubtedly true because of the timing.

It was the unusual feature of a severe and possibly mutilating skin disease, affecting solely the phallus which pointed to a psychic disturbance of considerable gravity. He it was who had given him the bicycle as a present. Although his relief at finding the child alive, and the subsequent hope that all would be well were both annulled, by the disappointment when he discovered the extent of the injuries, to his son. The expected future life of his child as an independent man was to die the instant he learned of the future prognosis, which sadly was confirmed during the passing years.

The hope of every parent is that the child will reach a healthy maturity and be permitted to lead an independent and productive life. This hope in the case of the patient was without the possibility of fulfilment in such circumstances. Indubitably there has been a participation mystique with the child, and probably an unconscious identification, for the father expressed his rage against the neighbour for his lack of concern for his son, after the accident, in a singularly personal manner.

The phallus is the male creative organ, and when it appears in dreams or fantasies it symbolizes creativity. The urethral orifice is the orificium urethrae and has the appearance of an eye. Indeed there is considerable mythological tradition associated with the urethra itself, which permits the discharge of urine and the expression of semen during sexual congress, in the physical body. When the urethra is damaged both of these functions may be disturbed or even obstructed. To micturate or void urine is to rid oneself of the waste products occasioned by the normal metabolism of the body, psychically it symbolizes the expression of one's deepest emotions or feelings. The secretion of semen is central to the physical act of creation. The Kabiri, those mighty dwarf gods were the children of the great mother goddess of Samothrace, in the Aegean sea, were all phallic beings. They were usually deformed in some way, lamed, misshapen or mutilated. Furthermore they had considerable associations with the criminal world. They represented powerful creative impulses. The whole phallic symbolism of the Kabiri is bound up with this creative force and in the psyche is an image of great potency.

The phallus in this instance was the symbol of the creative impulse carried by the living child. It is perhaps not out of place to suspect that the skin disorder of this man represented symbolically the death in his soul of the living creative image enfolded in the life of his child. The fact that it was the meatal orifice which was obliterated by the disease is itself significant. It was representative of his inability to see, that is understand, and express both his anger, and his guilt for he had given the bicycle to the child, as well as his impotence, which was felt in the psyche. The deep suffering of the soul was revealed through the organ of the skin, and its wisdom urged the acceptance of the tragic nature of his son's fate and of course, at the same time, his own.

THE MAN WHOSE SISTER RAN AWAY

A man of forty years with a serious attack of lichen planus, in which the entire body, including the scalp was involved, was referred for therapy. In view of the extensive nature of the condition it was decided to hospitalise him.

He was married, and his marriage it seemed was satisfactory. He was fond of his wife, and loved his children. By profession he was an accountant, and had through the years built up a successful practice. His first psychological function was sensation, and his attitude was introverted. He was of course quite unable to account for the sudden development of the skin rash and had no remembrance of any unusual event. It was only when he was directly questioned about his personal life that he had an immediate and total recall of its inception. He simply could not understand afterwards how he had forgotten such an important and unprecedented event which had befallen him six months earlier just prior to the appearance of the eruption. However the nature of the said event was quite compatible with its loss for it was indeed too painful for him to hold in consciousness.

The patient had a much beloved older sister, who like him was married with a family. Her husband was well respected in the town where they lived, and she herself, in her brother's description 'was an admirable woman'. Because her husband had a successful business she lived in very comfortable circumstances, and her children were able to attend good schools. Suddenly one afternoon without any warning whatever, this lady, believed by all to be a model wife suddenly disappeared. There was apparently no suspicions of illness, no evidence of mental instability, and she had exhibited nothing in the way of anxiety or depression in the preceding weeks, on the contrary she appeared to be happy and content.

The children had been seen off to school by their mother in the morning, and on return they found the house in good order, but the mother was absent. No note could be found, nor was there any rational explanation for her absence, such an event was out of keeping with her character. Eventually after an extensive police search had proved unsuccessful, the family was advised to wait. This led to severe anxieties on the part of the husband, and extreme trauma for the children. The great fear was that she had been murdered. In due course after some weeks of distress it was discovered that she was alive and living in the capital. She was apparently almost destitute and was greatly in need of money, which was the reason why she contacted her husband. It was decided that her brother, the patient should go to see her as he might be less emotional than the husband and therefore better equipped to deal with the situation.

The patient found his sister living in conditions of extreme squalor. The story which she gave to him, was as follows. Apparently out of boredom, she had started to go out in the afternoons to singles' bars in the town, where she drank, and met men, usually for an hour or so. It was during one of these such afternoons she met a man with whom she fell in love, and for whom she left home and family. It transpired that he was a violent criminal. He had served a prison sentence just before his meeting with the woman, but had in fact, served several terms in prison prior to this event. His record was a list of crimes of violence of different sorts.

When the patient found her, she begged for money which he gave her. He did not see the man, but during the following weeks she wrote regularly to her brother demanding considerable sums of money, both for herself and her lover. Gradually her condition worsened, she became a drug addict, and finally a thief. She was arrested and imprisoned. It was at this juncture the patient came for therapy. When he divulged the story of his sister's downfall he admitted that only his brother-in-law, and his own wife knew the full story, but these two were not told of the absolute degradation in which he found her, he kept this painful information to himself. She was literally in a state of starvation, there was neither food nor money in the place. She herself was unkempt, her clothes were torn and dirty, and she was bruised about the body. There were no creature comforts whatsoever in the hovel in which she was lodged. He did not at that time realize that she had become a drug addict, nor did he think of this added problem. He did consider however that she might have become insane.

During the time he spent with her, a great fear began to possess him also. At first he could not believe that the woman before him was his sister. Gradually during the days which followed he began to fear that he might go crazy himself. It was directly after he had met his sister that the lichen planus had begun to make its appearance, accompanied by ferocious irritation. The patient was still supporting his sister at the time of his admission to hospital, albeit she was in custody. He said he felt compelled to do so.

The first task was to reassure him that the episode was similar to a nightmare, and that although the reality of it could not be denied, he himself was not insane. This was accepted by him readily, and he was able to relax, with considerable alleviation of the general anxiety. It was then indicated to him that his sister was no longer his responsibility, and he was advised to discuss the whole matter frankly with his brother-in-law and his own wife. In due course he was able to understand that his sister had been caught by evil, which was the problem he had to face, and later to explain to her family. By this means eventually he was able to comprehend the great fear which had possessed him when he encountered his sister's transformation into total degradation.

It is unwise to make a conjectural assessment of the actual psychological condition of the sister without a direct confrontation. However from the facts presented, it seems that a quiet respectable practical woman, both wife and mother suddenly fell into her dark side and was possessed by the shadow. When she met the violent criminal, undoubtedly she came face to face with a hithertofore unknown aspect of her masculine unconscious. This inner dark animus was the instigator of the fatal attraction to the outer brutal and sadistic criminal. On the surface it would seem highly improbable that such a thing could happen. Here was a woman married to a well respected man with a kindly and decent brother who lived her life very comfortably, attending to the needs of her family. Possibly everything was well ordered, routinely easy and contained, no great expenditure of energy was required, and her outlook had become consequently, narrowed.

In such circumstances, unfortunately by no means uncommon for modern women, the animus finds a soil in which he can flourish like the green bay tree. He it is who becomes the whisperer, he begins to tell her that she is bored, not appreciated by her husband or children. He further tells her, she is getting old, perhaps she is missing something. Maybe her husband of many years has become jaded and the sexual act a routine duty. In this case the animus will have a great deal to say regarding the pleasures which may be found with other men, before it is too late. The inner voice of her dark companion seductively sweet, leads her to new ventures, alcoholism, particularly if there is a spiritual void in her life, drug addition, and sexual caprice to name the most frequent. Thus experimentation paves the way for the outer confrontation, which is the mirror image of the inner drama. In the case of this woman the seduction led to untold suffering not only for herself, but for her entire, immediate circle. Without thought of family, children, or friends she was swept away. She fell completely into her dark side, and all the virtues and values, appertaining to her former life were nullified. All that remained eventually was a poor physical wreck of the former woman.

The patient himself made a steady and relatively rapid recovery after he had begun to understand his sister's predicament and to relieve himself of the burden of her downfall. He decided to continue to attend regularly until his skin eruption had cleared. For over one year he slowly moved back to a state of normality, and in the end he made a satisfactory recovery.

At the end of this period he suddenly received the news that his sister had committed suicide, because it seemed, the criminal lover deserted her, after she was discharged from prison. The patient was able to weather the emotional storm subsequent to her death, without a further attack or exacerbation of the disease process.

The sister had already committed a psychic suicide when she left her family and her home to go with the sadistic criminal. The moment ego consciousness was possessed by the animus, she was lost, in effect she died then, the decent woman she had been before, succumbed. The brutal and sadistic animus was evident in her dealings with her loved ones. She left the house without warning, and the children returning from the school found it empty. She left no warning note of her departure, no intimation whatsoever of her whereabouts. Her family and her brother suffered many weeks of tortuous anxiety and dread for her welfare, not knowing whether she was alive or dead. Such an animus responsible for persuading her to behave thus, was the equivalent of the outer brutal sadist she met in reality. She encountered that fateful afternoon in the singles' bar her own dark inner masculine self of which she was totally unconscious. He had always been there waiting in the shadows, for the moment which he had so ably engineered, to make his presence felt. No one who knew her it seemed, could have suspected that she would fall into such misery, but such are the vicissitudes and strange dark interludes in life which belong to individual fate.

119

The lichen planus eruption which overwhelmed this man and gave to his skin the colour of a corpse was the harbinger of the death of his feeling for his sister. In a way he had already mourned her death when he found her in abysmal degradation in the capital. At the same time it was also a portent of his sister's eventual self-destruction. The skin buffered the fear he felt when he believed her insane, and feared that he himself was crazy. Madness is undoubtedly catching, and such fears are easily attracted in the company of psychotics. Thus the suffering occasioned by the illness was eventually to provide a psychic stability during the dark days when her death was made known to him. He had bravely and correctly ceased to support her and her lover, as soon as he realized she was no longer his responsibility, and he was not her keeper.

The skin indubitably was the reflector of the death of the light sister complex, and the loss of the fraternal feeling, in the realization of the dark shadow of his sister.

THE MAN WHOSE WIFE TRIED TO KILL HIM

Again in this case history, the death of a complex is observed. This was a man of sixty years of age, he had suffered an attack of severe lichen planus accompanied by overwhelming irritation, for which he required in-patient therapy. The symptom permitted him neither ease nor rest, and the condition had started eight months before. He himself was an extremely rational man and his superior function was thinking with an extraverted attitude. He knew exactly when the eruption had started and could give a clear account of its beginnings, moreover he knew why. He outlined the following story.

One night whilst sleeping by his wife's side, he was suddenly awakened from his sleep by a terrific blow to the chest. In that instant he was awake and saw his wife standing over him. In the darkness he caught the flash of a carving knife as it plunged into his chest for the second time. He realized that her hovering body which was looming over him was in the act of stabbing him. Before he was sufficiently awake, she succeeded in stabbing him four times in all. He was able to fend himself off and get out of the room to the telephone to call for help before he collapsed. His life was saved only by the fact that he lived close to a hospital. Within a very short period of time he was transfused with several pints of blood. One of the stab wounds had perforated the pericardium of the heart, the others had penetrated deep into the lungs.

The eruption of lichen planus appeared on the third day after the stabbing whilst he was in intensive care. He related it directly to the shock of the incident, which he had thought in the first instance was a dream. The rash persisted unchanged for eight months and was as mentioned accompanied by a severe furor dermaticus.

After the stabbing his wife was removed at once to a psychiatric hospital and was treated there for a matter of three weeks. The psychiatric departmental staff duly considered her condition at the end of this period, and it was decided that she should be discharged back to her home. At the same time a stipulation was made that the patient should give up his job, in order to look after his wife. As soon as he had recovered from the assault, and was pronounced fit to return to his home, he agreed to the proposal and affirmed that he would undertake her nursing care. He duly did so, and obtained a post as a night-security guard.

For a multiplicity of reasons, it was decided by the police authorities, the communal medical care workers, and the psychiatric medical advisors that proceedings would not be taken against the wife of the patient. Therefore she was not apprehended or subjected to any form of general public examination of her act. The psychiatrists in charge of the case made a diagnosis of myxoedema madness. Myxoedema is a condition whereby the thyroid gland becomes under-active. It is characterized by obesity, a dry skin with puffiness of the facies and lower limbs, and is accompanied by a condition of torpor, to a lesser or greater degree. Usually hypertension and heart disease are intervening factors.

The woman had been treated by her general practitioner for this condition, but had not received the specific therapy of thyroid extract. A complication which is described is one of episodic madness, and it is thought to be a sequel of this disease. It appears that the psychiatrists decided that since she appeared to be sane after she had been admitted to hospital and given thyroid extract, that the episode had been due to a sudden bout of lunacy, appertaining to her physical condition. Eventually she was discharged as normal, but requiring observant care. On arrival home she told her husband that she was sorry, and he said that he forgave her. When he was asked why the case appeared to have been dealt with in an unusual way, he said he would rather not discuss it, it was all too painful for him. It was however pointed out to him that there seemed to have been a miscarriage of justice, but that for him was an unacceptable assumption.

But from the moment of his return to his home, after his own recovery, he decided to take the job as a night guard and during the day would only sleep in the house if a woman relative was there to look after his wife. At the same time that he returned home, he found that he had become impotent. During the period whilst he was undergoing therapy for the lichen planus he stated repeatedly, that it would have been a terrible thing if his wife had gone to prison, or entered a mental hospital. He said many times, that the psychiatrists were kind, and had looked after his wife so admirably. It was eventually indicated to him, that he was afraid to sleep in the house with his wife. At first he denied this. It was then intimated that the fact that he was impotent was a further barrier against his sleeping with his wife.

Eventually he was persuaded to look at the facts, and as a rational man, he was able to do so, there was the night employment the woman relative as guardian whilst he was sleeping, and the impotency. Still he would not admit that he was afraid of his wife.

Then he developed urticaria. As seen previously urticaria is a condition, associated with intense irritation of the skin, accompanied by blotches. The word urticaria is derived from the Latin word for nettle, urticare. When urticaria intervenes it is exactly as if one has fallen into a bed of nettles. The skin exhibits angry red welts described as weals, and the urticated lesions move from one part of the body to another. As stated, the appearance of the skin resembles nothing so much as a smouldering heath fire, which blazes up and dies down, only to recommence in another venue. The skin exactly mirrors the underlying emotional fires which blaze, smoulder, flare up and die away, only to return again to the unconscious.

When it was suggested to the patient that perhaps he was really very angry with the whole situation because he no longer had peace of mind and metaphorically speaking had in fact already fallen into a bed of nettles, at last he agreed and he admitted that he was mortally afraid of his wife. He was advised to visit the psychiatrist in charge of his wife's case, but he refused, he was then advised to seek psychiatric advice elsewhere, but he could not entertain the re-opening of the case, and he declined.

The main reason for his reluctance was that he was unable to bear the guilt of hospitalizing his wife. He knew that she was psychotic, and later admitted that she had had strange, even bizarre episodes some of an unusual nature before, but she had never physically attacked him. Strangely the fact of her murderous impulse was never considered in totalis, the psychiatric advices were less than reasonable in the circumstances. His position was not considered, and therefore became untenable and unbearable. Most certainly he was a rational thinking type and feeling was his inferior function. He was quite divorced from his inner and instinctual nature. He knew of course that his wife was physically ill, but he had not realized her depressions and occasional bizarre behaviour held any danger for him. His previous occupation dealt mostly with the criminal world, and it appeared that he had accustomed himself to this world and accepted certain standards not conducive for his own well being. After the stabbing he was smitten with deep fear, but he was so alienated from his instinctual self that he did not recognise his own terror. He believed he had loved his wife and continued to protect her as a duty, but in his heart, he no longer had any positive feelings for her. He had not therefore visualized the reality of the situation and could not consciously grasp it. He had missed death by a hair's breadth, and his wife was a potential murderess, for she had raised the knife four times against her husband, and for which act she had not been publicly censored.

The lichen planus exhibited the death of his confidence, it certainly pointed to an inner death of the love for his wife. It remained as long as he denied his terror, and his real feelings. The remarkable fact that the urticaria supervened, accentuated the need for him to face his inner emotional disturbance, and become aware of it. When urticaria is visible on the skin the ephemeral nature of its ebb and flow, always appears to indicate a potential, and frequently impending acceptance of emotional reaction hithertofore unrecognised by the subject.

The patient in this case had repressed the reality of the horrifying event, he had not permitted himself to remember it and by the same token, had no consciousness of the accompanying emotions, chiefly terror and rage with underlying hatred for the wife. The emotions thus left to their own devices increased in intensity. Undoubtedly the first skin reaction of lichen planus revealed the profundity and the magnitude of the emotion in the unconscious, then followed urticaria which was infinitely more distressing for him, but which was the means by which he was forced to realize the truth.

THE MAN WHO LOST HIS MOTHER

A farmer of forty-seven years of age presented with a severe lichen planus affecting only the mouth. The reaction extended throughout the mucous surface of the oral cavity, and along the line of the vermilion border of both the upper and lower lips. The entire mouth was etched out as with an indelible red pencil, therefore the gaze was directed only towards the mouth, and the rest of the face, appeared at first to be a nondescript blur. The impression received was that the mouth which had been forced open by the swelling of the tissues, had been frozen in the position of a silent cry.

He was unmarried and was the eldest of a family of several children. The father had been a farmer, but had died when the man himself was only sixteen years of age. The burden of the farm had fallen upon these young shoulders, as had the upbringing of the younger brothers and sisters. The widowed mother was an able woman, but she looked to the eldest son in all matters of importance, so that in the end he became her staunch supporter, as well as the provider for the family for the rest of his life.

The lichen planus started within a month of his mother's death. He related the event of her death as being causative of the condition. Apparently he had been her sole companion for a number of years, as all the other children left home either to marry or take up careers. In his own words he said that "he missed her, but he realized that she had an incurable illness some months previously and had prepared himself for her death". After the funeral, and the departure of the mourners, he suddenly found that he was quite alone. His farm was isolated high on a moorland area at a considerable distance from a town.

It was, it seemed efficiently run, and he had plenty of time for leisure, but alas because of his situation he suddenly found himself without friends, or interests. He was very amiable, and a particularly pleasant person, but there was always a suspicion that he was close to panic. In his conversation this was revealed by the odd or chance remark in which he asked a question about his future health, or futurity as such. Unfortunately he produced no dreams, and as the months passed, very little progress was made. Eventually it was decided to approach the question of his mother's death in more detail. Then and only then, about six months after he had first presented himself, did it become clear that his relationship with his mother had been far from ideal. He had totally suppressed his real feelings and in fact for over thirty years had been dominated by her. She had put him in his father's place, and then proceeded to disallow any freedom of movement in any direction, other than the actual organization of the farm, which through the years he accomplished in fine style. This man was of an exceedingly agreeable nature, and he had permitted himself to be tyrannised by his mother, because he felt that she had had a hard life. In a sense he had come to disregard his own wishes, feelings, and sexuality and always deferred to the desire of his mother. He explained that he had never spoken against her in his life.

As he was able to express himself the brutal plum colour of his mouth began to abate, and the lichen planus begun slowly to heal. It was interesting that psyche chose the mouth to express itself at last.

An interesting development in this case was that at long last when he was able to permit himself to speak the truth of his relationship with his parent, an unsuspected talent erupted. He suddenly found that he could not only draw and paint, but that he could do so, surprisingly well. Within a year or so he retired from his farming occupational activities, and seriously took up his new metier. It is in retrospect evident that the domination of the mother archetype in its negative form had obstructed the inner spring of creativity. As a farmer he had developed his practical and feeling side, but the inferior function of intuition was to bloom in the singularly imaginative paintings. This was therefore the expression necessary for his individuation and could only come into being by way of the curious development of the oral lichen planus.

His soul selected the lips to speak a silent language, in which he was to learn that the false attachment to his mother was no more and at the death of the lie, the new creative life could be born.

REFERENCES

1 Blum, Richard and Eva, The Dangerous Hour, Love and Culture Crisis in Ancient Greece.

8

ALOPECIA AREATA AND TOTALIS (LOSS OF HAIR, CIRCUMSCRIBED AND TOTAL)

This condition in which discrete patches of baldness appear on the scalp, accounts for two per cent of all new dermatological out-patient attendances in the United Kingdom and the United States.[1] Macalpine[2] states "Some investigators consider that emotional factors play no significant rôle in alopecia areata" whereas Feldman[3] claims that most patients are psychologically abnormal. The general conclusion however in dermatological circles is that alopecia areata is not a psychosomatic disorder.

Alopecia areata arises usually without evidence of local disease. It consists of a single patch or patches of denuded skin clearly defined and symptomless. It tends to recover satisfactorily but does often recur. In severe cases, there is sometimes a total hair loss.

It may be also that the entire body hair disappears. If the scalp hair is lost in totalis it can still recover, but frequently does not, and then the baldness is permanent. In these cases the sufferer comes to resemble a newly born baby.

It has always been thought that a great many such cases are attributable to a severe shock. This is indubitably true, but there is usually an added factor. For example, an eight year old girl visited her aunt regularly after school, one day she found her brutally murdered in the kitchen of her home. The child lost all the scalp hair within ten days of witnessing this horrifying sight. However, the woman unbeknown, of course, to the child and her family had been a prostitute. This fact entailed a necessary and detailed questioning of the child by the authorities in an effort to discover the killer. The reaction of the family and friends to this uncovered scandal, also had a profound effect upon the child.

A woman woke up one morning and discovered that during the night her hair had fallen out, and she was quite bald. Because of the rhythmic nature of hair growth it was enquired of her whether anything unusual had occurred, three months earlier. She could not recall anything untoward and indeed forgot, until reminded by her husband, that she had visited her brother's home which was abroad, three months earlier. Furthermore she had also forgotten that whilst there a particularly shocking event occurred. During supper one evening, the hostess, the woman's sister-in-law got up from the table and went to the kitchen. She returned at once, with a carving knife, and plunged it into her husband's back. Fortunately he survived, with expert care, the wife was committed for psychiatric therapy, and the patient was very shocked. The experience was too distressing for her to retain in consciousness. It is not difficult to perceive the relationship between the two events. The woman was required however to retain the event in ego consciousness, and to bear the suffering enfolded in the knowledge.

A young boy of seven years lost all his hair at the age of four years, and it had never regrown. His physical appearance was that of a new born baby, with a round chubby face and smooth hairless head. He was quiet and timid, and spoke little. His father was loud, uncouth, and dominating. The mother was unsympathetic towards the child, afraid no doubt to displease the father. Whilst the parents were engaged in conversation during the consultation it was deemed advisable to send the child to the waiting room to draw. Meanwhile the mother corroborated the father's statement that the child was not nervous, frightened or emotional. She could think of no reason why the child had lost his hair. The boy returned with a pencil drawing. The image was simple, it consisted of a fair sized house which was just in the act of exploding at the precise moment that it was hit by a bomb released from an overhead war plane. When asked whose house it was, the child said, "Mummy and Daddy's!" (be it noted not 'mine'). The father said "It is only a child's drawing!". The child had spoken via the image, it was the parents who required therapy.

Finally to continue with the theme of 'forgetting' the following patient is recalled to mind. She was a beautiful woman who looked perhaps twenty-five years of age. She was in fact in her fifties.

She had a smooth unlined face, perfect contours, flawless maquillage a full head of hair, thin pencilled eye-brows, and curled synthetic eye-lashes. She had come to enquire whether there was any up to date therapy because she had been completely bald for thirty years, of both scalp and body hair. Without the wig which she was wearing an extraordinary transformation took place. In a twinkling of an eye she at once assumed the appearance of a slightly weathered newly born baby.

She had been married for twenty years to a much older man who was also extremely rich. She had twin daughters of nineteen years, and her life was passed in considerable comfort between her homes in Europe and the

Mediterranean. She denied that she had suffered an illness or shock at the time of the onset of the disorder. She could venture no opinion as to why she should have lost her hair. There was little point in pursuing this line of thought as to the cause, since the event had occurred so long ago.

The following two years were devoted to courses of various therapies, without avail, and she was told that nothing further could be done. A year later she returned because of ill health. I decided to refer her to a cardiologist. He discovered, during the course of his examination, a small scar under the left breast. She told him that it was a bullet wound. When next I saw her I enquired as to its presence.

She had forgotten to tell me the details of an incident which occurred when she was nineteen years old, thirty years before. At the time she was engaged to be married to a serving soldier. Just prior to the wedding her mother advised her not to marry the young man. She explained that since the father's death by accident, the previous year, the family fortune was in jeopardy. The mother considered the young man to be too poor, and not a good match for her daughter. The following evening the dutiful daughter went out with her fiancée and quite simply told him what her mother had advised. Not unnaturally he was very upset. Eventually at his insistence she agreed to meet again the following evening for a last dinner together. The fiancée called for her in his motor car. He pleaded once more for her to change her mind. She refused, so he drew his pistol and he shot her in the motor car. The bullet lodged in the wall of the heart, and fortunately did not penetrate the chamber. She was unconscious for a week, and then she recovered. In that week she lost all her hair and it never grew again.

When enquiries were made regarding the fate of the young man, she said that she thought he had gone to prison but she had no idea of his eventual fate.

She had completely forgotten this incident until the cardiologist saw the scar. She had never told her husband or her children. She had put away this dreadful secret. The story was related to me with a quiet and smiling composure, and the overall appearance was eminently suggestive of a beautiful innocent child of perhaps three years of age. This was probably her emotional age.

Undoubtedly she had a close call and had been within a hair's breadth of death. The soldier had meant to kill her. His reaction was certainly unforgiveable but in the circumstances, understandable. She virtually plunged a knife into the man's heart, when she quoted her mother, he retaliated in the same vein, and wounded hers.

Behind this catastrophe there is the mother. Here indeed is a very dark feminine consciousness, she disregarded her daughter as an individual, no enquiry was made as to her feelings for the boy, no thought given to the boy himself. Possessed by power the mother decided. That decision was in fact the act which set in motion the chain of events which culminated in the firing of the pistol. The daughter was an insipid pawn in the game caught in the cocoon of the mother archetype, without consciousness of herself as a woman.

Reflection did not follow the shooting, the woman herself gave no thought to the question of provocation, her conception of her own rôle in the drama was unsullied by doubt. Ego consciousness could not assimilate the burden of knowledge, so she retreated from the purgatorial fire of consciousness of the event. She preferred to remain as she was, the child of her mother, or the slave of the maternal animus. The night she followed her mother's advice was a fateful one, almost a fatal one. Since the feminine ego consciousness was not increased she was not able to disengage herself from her mother's opinions, nor was she any nearer to becoming conscious of herself as a woman. She continued to live for thirty years in the same unconscious state, dutifully living out her mother's unlived life. But at what cost? Her unlined, beautiful childlike face, and the hairless head, bore the stamp of the avoidance of conscious awareness, and its entailed suffering . . .

THE SPELLBOUND WOMAN

This was a woman in her forties who presented in a very unusual way. Her doctor telephoned me to say that she had lost her hair, but she also complained that she had a snake curled up in the centre of her back. He believed that she was crazy. As he spoke to me on the telephone, I had a sudden vision of the Kundalini serpent. When she arrived, she confirmed all that the doctor had described. Except, in spite of her strange statement regarding the serpent I did not suspect a psychosis,

The anamnesis revealed that she was originally from the Mediterranean region, but had lived in northern Europe for many years. Her two children were both adolescent, and the family had been very content and happy until her husband met a young woman, with whom he had a sexual affair. The girl became pregnant, and he decided to leave his wife and children for the girl. The wife, as a staunch catholic woman refused to divorce him. An uneasy truce appeared, but was shattered during the early hours of one morning.

The husband not having returned home from work the wife and children retired to bed. During the early hours of the following morning, the woman woke up and found that she had great difficulty in breathing, she realized that the gas fire was turned on, but unlit, she managed to go to the windows, and open them. With great difficulty she crawled to the children's rooms, and found that there was a similar situation. Both the children were unconscious, but their mother sought help at once, and their lives were saved.

The drama had in fact only begun for it was discovered that the husband had returned to the house, and entered quietly turning on all the gas taps in the upstair's rooms. He had then departed with his woman friend. He was caught by the police and tried for attempted murder, receiving a prison sentence.

Within three weeks of the attempt on her life, the woman's hair began to fall. It was then she became aware of the snake in her back. She explained that if the snake moved upwards, the hair would grow. I asked her what was the colour of the snake, and she told me it was black.

Slowly over the succeeding months, she began to improve in general health. The hair began to regrow, and after it had reached the length of about three inches, in six months it once again fell. This cycle was repeated at least twice more. At the end of two years, I asked her if the snake in her back had gone, she told me that it was still there. However she then burst into tears, and said that every night for the previous seven months she had had the same dream. She was so afraid, that she could hardly sleep at all. But at whatever time she went to sleep, the dream always awakened her,

A repetitive dream always signifies a content of the utmost importance in the unconscious, which is urging for self realization. I asked her to tell me the dream, and she described it as follows.

"I am sleeping in my own bed, in my room, in the bed I used to sleep in, with my husband. The room is light, because the door is open, and there standing on the threshold of the room in the open door is my mother-in-law, looking at me, and holding out her hands with the palms towards me."

I asked her if she could tell me anything about her mother-in-law. She answered quite simply. "She is a witch." Since this is a not uncommon expression used to describe mothers-in-law, I asked for more details. The patient answered, that the mother-in-law really was a witch, she contended that she earned her living as a practising witch in a Mediterranean country, and was able to achieve all kinds of bewitchment of persons and animals, because of her skilled sorcery. She was it seemed well known, in the area where she lived. Since the dream had occurred nightly for over half a year, a further exploration of the woman's background was undertaken.

It came to light that she had been a girl of simple, exceedingly poor but devout peasant family.

The most powerful family in the area had a son who was to fall in love with the patient. When they decided to marry the boy's mother, the sorceress, was against the union and did all she could to prevent it. In the end the young couple eloped, and went to live abroad where they married. The patient said that in all the subsequent years, her mother-in-law neither accepted nor forgave her.

Apparently the dream was very vivid, and the gesture of the mother-in-law's hands, with exposed palms, signified in the patient's view, a curse. I saw no reason to disbelieve her and decided to consult the priest of her parish church, where she worshipped. With her permission I told the priest of the dream, since she had not thought to confess its repeated presence to him. There seemed little doubt that the question of evil was paramount, the

129

woman was bewitched. But what to do? It became evident, considering the background of the woman, her beliefs, her fears and general status that the only course available was to seek a neutralization of the bewitched state, and thereby save her soul. It simply was not possible to undertake an analysis, so other means were explored. It is not easy today to discover the whereabouts of an exorcist in modern Europe. After fruitless search the priest suggested that he should perform the blessing of the baptismal ceremony himself.

As a rite of initiation or consecration, this ceremony enfolds a multitude of events, associated with initiatory rites, water symbolism, and immersion, for it belongs to the world of myth and folk lore and superstitions, in which lies the foundations of all religious beliefs. The baptismal font as the benedictio fontis is the womb of the church.

"In the ceremony known as the benedictio fontis the baptismal font is apostrophised as 'immaculatus divini fontis uterus' the immaculate womb of the divine font".[4] Jung adds "the holy water has salt put into it with the idea of making it like amniotic fluid or sea water."[5] In the Christian church the baptistry was separated from the main body of the building because it was a mystery place. Originally the font of the church was a piscina, a pond in which the initiates were immersed to be bathed, which was in fact a symbolic drowning. It was believed that after the metaphoric death they emerged from the bath of baptism as a transformed being, quasi modi geniti, the reborn.

Therefore as Jung[6] explains "the crypt or baptismal font has the meaning of a place of terror and death and also of rebirth, a place where dark initiations take place".

The Christian sacrament of baptism signifies a marker of the most singular importance in the psychic development of the human race. Jung[7] says:

> "Baptism endows the individual with a living soul. I do not mean that the baptismal rite in itself does this, by a unique and magical act. I mean that the idea of baptism lifts man out of his archaic identification with the world and transforms him into a being who stands above it. The fact that mankind has risen to the level of this idea is baptism in the deepest sense, for it means the birth of the spiritual man, who transcends nature."

The priest's suggestion was taken up, and he duly performed the ceremony. The change in the patient was remarkable. The dream did not recur again, and slowly after about a year, she lost her fears, and was able to live a relatively peaceful life. Her hair regrew within the subsequent two years, and did not fall again. However, quite by chance she remarked that the snake was still there, but it had moved to a higher level. It was originally in the small of the back, at the level of the sacro-iliac joints. After its ascension, it was situated at the level of the 4th and 5th dorsal vertebrae, in the centre of the upper back. It was about this time that she proposed to visit the country of her birth. She decided that she would also visit one of the world's greatest churches to give prayers of thanksgiving.

Since she was going to be in the immediate vicinity of the sorceress I suggested that it might be expedient for her to undergo a second and expert exorcism at the same time. To serve so to speak as a protective safeguard against the proximity of the fire.

In due course she returned to see me and declared that she had visited a prince of the catholic church, to whom she had divulged all that which had befallen her. He received her confession, and gave the blessing. However when she told him of my suggestion regarding an expert exorcism as a protection against the witch, he told her it was not necessary. He added that there are no longer any witches!

The question of the black serpent remained, and gave me cause for uneasiness. Her hair had regrown, and was abundant, her spirits had lifted and it seemed that she had recovered.

A black snake signifies, darkness, death, invisibility and unconsciousness. The movement upwards signified a subjective experience of an unconscious content, far removed from consciousness, rising slowly towards the possibility of assimilation, and increase of conscious awareness.

The fundamental idea of Tantric Yoga is that a feminine creative force in the shape of a serpent named Kundalini rises up from the perineal centre where she has been sleeping and ascends through the chakras activating them and constellating their symbols. This power, is called the serpent power, a force which is personified as a goddess called Mahadevishakti. She signifies the one who is able to bring everything into existence, for which she uses maya, the building material of reality. The fourth chakra of the ascension of Kundalini is Anahata, and it is situated in the region of the heart and diaphragm, which corresponds to the mid-dorsal region of the spinal column, posteriorly. It represents the seat of feeling and thinking.

The serpent also is the god of healing and at the same time it contains wisdom and prophecy.

At last I decided to ask her what still gave her cause for concern. She denied any difficulties, with a slight shrug. A year afterwards she became depressed and it transpired that her husband, soon to be released from prison, wished to marry the woman who was the mother of his child. The patient refused, because as a catholic she would not contemplate divorce. Undoubtedly she was a practising catholic, and most certainly a devout woman. It became apparent to me that the snake represented an unconscious feeling or thought which pressed towards conscious acceptance. Whilst married to the man who had wished to murder her, there was still a tie. Moreover, his mother the sorceress, represented the maternal aspect of his anima. Somewhere in the shadow of the patient there was also a witch. She had been gripped by an idea which alienated her from her true

131

self, and she was thus dissociated. The backbone represents the will, she had a will as powerful as her sorceress mother-in-law. She was determined to keep her husband from re-marrying, not simply because it was against the edict of the church, but for revenge. I suggested that she thought further about divorce, but she was adamant. The secret wish was that if as her rightful husband he did not want her, she would see that he would never belong to another. This wish emanates from the deepest strata of the instinctual feminine realm, where human nature and that of the animal are as one.

In retrospect the whole drama had hinged on this fact. It was highly significant that the unconscious spoke to her, through the medium of the hair, a woman's crowning glory. Its loss gave her the appearance of a newly born babe. This was the image of potential transformation of her attitude which was waiting to take place. Only a partial transformation occurred, one which conformed exactly with the collective. It was enough to permit her hair, representative of thoughts to regrow. Thus the snake represented an invisible obstruction in her process of individuation. It was then she decided to leave my care, and I did not see her again.

RESUMÉ

The material of these reports reveals in all, the archetype of murder, a not infrequent finding in my experiences in cases of alopecia; particularly the totalis type.

In the case of the boy who drew the parental home, the child's psyche was a reflection of that of his parents. The father was bombastic, and had a coarse and brutal shadow. The wife, as the mother of the child was without Eros, and totally unsupportive of the child. The fact that the hair had grown, and then disappeared, indicates a severe regression of libido. The urgent realization of himself as a personage, an individual was indicated by the hair loss. He was required to be reborn, to grow up to an awareness of his own self, distinct from the father and mother. If the atmosphere of the home is psychologically unhealthy, as was the case with this boy, the child's psychic equilibrium is destabilized. There is a tremendous natural urge to life and a deep contact with the life instinct in children. It is this latter which urges towards healthy adjustment. This is the meaning behind the development of alopecia in this child. Psychological therapy for the parents would have been the answer for the child, but there was no possibility of this.

With the case of the little girl, undoubtedly there was considerable knowledge on the child's side as regards the aunt's occupation. However this was concealed, except for one or two seemingly innocent remarks. The extreme reaction of her parents, with the publicity at school, upset the child, but also accentuated deep feelings of guilt, stemming from the actual relationship of the woman and the child.

The woman who witnessed the stabbing was required to increase her consciousness regarding the married life of her brother and his wife. The brutal nature of the attempted murder was hastily forgotten, but the unconscious did not allow this, consciousness was required, together with insight into the causes. The other two cases, both concerned with attempted murder were remarkable each in its own way for the degree of unconsciousness present, and the resistance to enlightenment.

In all, the presence of real evil is evident. Jung is often quoted as using the dictum of Christ, "Except ye become little children". To become children again, means to return to the realm of childhood, so that one may grow up in order to leave it to become adult, aware of the problem of evil in the world. One stays in the land of innocence at one's peril.

REFERENCES

1 Rook, A., Wilkinson, D. S., Ebling, F. J. G., Textbook Dermatology, Vol. 11, p. 1777, Published Blackwell.
2 Macalpine, I., 1958, British Journal of Dermatology, 1. para 70, 117.
3 Feldman, M., Rondon, H. A. J., (1975) Med. Cut. 7. 95.
4 Jung, C. G., Collected Works, Vol. 7, para 171, Routledge & Kegan Paul, London.
5 Ibid., Vol. 8, para 336.
6 Ibid., Vol. 18 para 256.
7 Ibid., Vol. 10 para 136.

9

THE VESICULAR (BLISTERING) DISEASES
Dermatitis Herpetiformis

INTRODUCTION

This distressingly irritating disease is benign, recurrent and chronic. It presents itself with an eruption enfolding features of redness, urtication, and blistering. Men are affected twice as frequently as women, and the adult form can be found in children. It occurs most commonly between the ages of twenty to fifty-five years. The blister is sited subepidermally at the level between the basal lamina and the dermis.

THE INITIATION OF A BOY INTO MANHOOD

A young man of seventeen years suddenly became gravely ill. Twenty-four hours before he had been completely well, but after complaining of a slight feverishness he had gone to bed, and in the morning it was discovered that his entire body from head to foot was covered in blisters. During the day, he became increasingly confused, developing a high pyrexia, and the blisters later became haemorrhagic.

He lived in a country district, and his general practitioner was very disturbed by the sight of the eruption, together with the pyrexia and semi-comatose condition of the boy. In those days, there was still the serious possibility of smallpox, either due to foreign travel, or laboratory contact with infected material. The doctor used a textbook of dermatology to make the diagnosis, and decided that it was smallpox, albeit the patient did not work in a laboratory nor had he been abroad. When I was asked to see him, I sympathized with the diagnosis, but the question of smallpox fortunately did not arise.

134

In due course after admission to a special hospital he was eventually diagnosed as a case of acute onset dermatitis herpetiformis. The original eruption had immediately given way to generalised blister formation, and had become intensely irritating. In an endeavour to relieve himself, and ease this grave symptom, he had literally torn himself to pieces. This fact partly accounted for the subsequent haemorrhagic nature of the blisters. From the day of admission to hospital, almost a year was to elapse before he was able to return home. The skin continued to erupt throughout most of this time, and occasional bouts of unexplained fever, would return for several days, and then just as quickly pass away. The young man was still at school having just taken the entrance examination to university, in fact he was awaiting the result of which, at the time the eruption began on his body.

Once the diagnosis was established and his parents and family reassured that there was no question of smallpox, therapy was instituted. All the usual and common therapeutic agents were tried but to no avail. The pyrexia was eventually controlled by various antibiotic agents, but the continued rhythmical appearance of blisters remained unchanged. After several months of effort, a combination of steroid therapy and dimethylsulphone produced a beneficial effect. The latter drug was in fact subsequently prescribed to the young man for over a decade and permitted him to live a comparatively trouble-free existence in spite of the continued presence of the disease.

The outstanding feature of the disorder was the multiplicity of large tightly packed oval blisters, which covered the body in a precise symmetrical fashion, so that the appearance of the two halves of the body were mirror images of each other. As the blisters erupted, the combination of itching, and scratching produced a blood-stained fluid which caused the body to be covered with a film which dried hard like lacquer. Consequently he was in extreme discomfort all the time, and frequently suffered considerable pain. After the first three months the life force re-asserted itself and it became apparent that the boy was going to recover.

He was highly intelligent, very personable, and throughout the illness was possessed of a high degree of courage. One outstanding feature of his personality was his obedience, often a very necessary virtue in times of severe illness. He complied with all instructions, and bravely bore the most painful and tedious ministrations.

When it became clear that death was not going to occur, a strange period of stasis resulted. Days passed, and no change occurred in his physical condition which reached a kind of plateau. Lesions appeared, reached a peak, erupted, dried and disappeared, only to reappear in the same fashion. A photographic record at the time revealed an unchanging rhythm over a period of several months. Since the mental attitude on the part of the boy began to improve it was decided to enquire further into the events which preceded the début, of this atrocious malady.

The story which unfolded revealed that prior to its onset, he had been very carefree and lighthearted having finished his examinations in which he felt he had acquitted himself admirably, an assumption which proved to be correct.

The school which he attended was co-educational and a party of young people had decided to celebrate Midsummer's Eve by going to the top of a nearby mountain to witness the sunrise of Midsummer's Day. The patient accompanied his friends and spent the night in their company. He returned for breakfast and was greeted by his mother who had waited up for him all night, seated in a chair, watching the door. In describing the events the boy said that his mother was "absolutely furious". Apparently he was quite unable to give her any kind of explanation as she would not listen, so caught was she in her anger. Three days later he awoke, and found that his body was covered with blisters. His mother thought that he had chickenpox a reasonable assumption, from the initial appearance. She waited a few days until his condition began to deteriorate, and then she called the doctor, who in turn thought it was smallpox.

After this first discussion, the boy and I were able to establish a very good rapport. From that time we regularly discussed the conditions at home, and what emerged is as follows.

His parents were both from the town in which the family lived, and were eminently respectable, and also well respected. The father was a business-man, and the mother stayed at home to look after their three sons. She was undoubtedly the driving force in the family. Scholastically the three chil-dren fulfilled her aim in that they acquitted themselves well at school, the older children were both at university. The patient who was the youngest son, was the favourite. About the time I began to examine the background of the case, the ward sister informed me that the mother had made a seri-ous complaint against the nursing staff. She accused a particular nurse of giving the boy pornographic literature. What had transpired was that the mother had visited him and found that he was reading a book which she considered to be erotic. A detailed investigation was undertaken and it was discovered that the book was simply a modern somewhat risqué novel by a best selling popular author, but, and this was the sting in the tail of the scorpion, the mother herself had brought the book in a parcel of reading material, for him.

This piece of enlightening information led the boy and I to an examina-tion of the motive behind the mother's accusation. At the end of our dis-cussion, the boy said "But she is like that all the time". In fact a turning point had been reached. He was to remain a further four months in hospi-tal and even though much improved at the time of discharge his skin was still severely affected. Throughout the subsequent three years whilst he was at university he continued to visit me. He took his medicaments regularly and he obtained a most presentable degree. During his last year at univer-sity he was invited by a friend to visit a foreign country. Later he told me that the moment he arrived there the dermatitis herpetiformis cleared, and he did not have a moment's discomfort during the six weeks he remained in that country. As soon as he returned to the country of his birth the eruption returned, but it was never as severe again as it had been originally. I asked him then if he loved his mother. The question caught him unawares, and he said "she is a good woman, and means very well, but I cannot love her, she restricts me".

Some years later he got a job abroad, and his dermatitis cleared, never to return. He married and became a successful businessman, having entered the business world instead of the academic life his mother had chosen and planned for him.

This skin disease can and does drive some of its victims to suicide because of the extraordinary degree of irritation which may arise. It came to the young man as an outer manifestation of a monumental inner conflict. He was of a rational extraverted personality, and his excellent thinking was his superior function. He had a well developed practical side, but feeling was inferior. He had lived a narrow secluded life confined to a small country town. His family belonged to a particularly narrow sect of the protestant faith and was devoted to church activities, and the members were all regular church goers. The church itself was the centrum of their lives.

The mother was a woman held to be possessed of many virtues, by her family and friends. She never raised her voice, and on the occasions that I met her, I saw no evidence of emotional display, not even at the onset of her son's illness when I had to inform her that there appeared to be a very real possibility that he might die. Undoubtedly as we have seen, she had a furious temper, but she gave the impression of coldness and distance and was singularly repellant. Her conversation revealed the presence of, indeed the possession by, a narrow rigid and intrusive animus, with the propensity to dominate a conversation. It seemed that her superior function was sensation which allowed her to be eminently practical and managing, and her attitude was introverted, this left her with intuition as her inferior function.

Clearly she had become dissociated from her inner instinctual world. The inferior function is the door through which all the figures of the unconscious come into consciousness. The inferior function is so close to the unconscious and is so undeveloped and barbarous, that it is the weak spot in consciousness in which the mighty figures of the unconscious can break in. The animus is the unconscious masculine personality of a woman, and carries all those thoughts and convictions, which belong to the masculine world, encountered by the woman in her life, and which are not necessarily her own as a feminine being.

Jung applied the term of animus to the inner face which in a woman is presented to the unconscious, whereas the 'outward face' or the persona is the face presented towards the reality world. The mother of this boy presented a face of chilling respectability and reserved withdrawal. Yet, in conversa-

137

tion one was conscious of a thrusting, bullying over-riding masculine force. This was her animus. If one can visualize the animus as it emerged into her consciousness through the open door of inferior intuition it is not difficult to understand the hideous, negative intuitive thoughts which seized her, and the barbarous imaginative fancies undoubtedly of a sexual nature which overwhelmed her on the night her son did not return. The opinions and her inferior intuition were apparent in the accusations against the pretty nurse and her negative erotic projections regarding the episode of the book. All of these incidents reveal how threatened she was, when her dearest possession, her third son was escaping from her, slipping from her grasp into manhood.

I had the impression in her icy composure, that the streams of her emotional life ran very deep indeed. I also perceived that when her emotional composure was breached, the furies would be insatiable, in their intent, This woman had a very dark shadow, of which she was completely unconscious. The illness of the young man was no less than that of the initiation into his consciousness of his mother's darkness, and it was this awareness which enabled him to become in the fullest sense of the word, a man. His masculine qualities of resilience, and courage, together with his obedience, learned with pain no doubt, through the years with his mother, enabled him to pursue the goal of health, which came with his own wholeness, and escape from his mother's world.

The principle factor in this strange story is the setting of the prologue to the drama, the place was the mountain, and the time was Midsummer's Eve.

From time immemorial throughout the whole of western Europe in an area stretching from Ireland in the west to Russia in the east, Scandinavia in the north, south to the Mediterranean sea, the eve of Midsummer's day has held an awesome significance for the ancestral minds of our fore-fathers.

It is difficult for modern man to comprehend the singular importance of these great fire festivals or to realize how widespread they were. One's knowledge is patchy but it seems that Midsummer's Eve was anciently the time of the Summer solstice, June 21st, later it became celebrated as it is today on June 23rd. In Christian times, this ancient Druidic festival has been termed the feast of St. John the Baptist, and today in Europe June 23rd is celebrated as St. John's Eve.

In times past it was customary on that day for the people of the hamlets and the villages of all the peasant communities, and later also in the towns to meet together and light midsummer fires at the tops of mountains, or hills. These fires played a tremendous rôle, cattle driven through them were cured of disease, dances and prayers performed around them, were to aid the crops to grow, and cause the rain to fall. There was also an element of romanticism, liaisons formed at these festivals, were dependent upon which of the young boys would remain faithful? Who would propose marriage? Who would not? Above all the bonfires were to ensure the farmers against the arts of witches, who stole the milk from the cows by means of spells.

138

In parts of Germany, young men who had lit the bonfires went from house to house and received jugfuls of milk.

It was also the practice to take home a lighted brand from the new fire and with it, rekindle the fire on the domestic hearth. It is clear that in interpreting the meaning of these great ubiquitous fire festivals one must review the universal customs attached, since all over Europe the traditional acts occurred. One is led to the conclusion that on the principle of imitative magic the fires may be regarded as sun charms to ensure sunshine in plenty for men, animals, and plants by kindling fires which mimic the sun as source of light and heat. This is the solar theory of Mannhardt.[1]

But on the other hand the fires have been regarded as the essential feature of purification rites. (This is a view held by Westermenck.[2]) Fire like sunshine is a creative power, providing warmth and light, but also is a destructive power which blasts and consumes, the fire is therefore stimulant and purifying. Undoubtedly the aim as regards the purification theory was to destroy or neutralize the skills of witchcraft, to protect men, crops and herds. Our forebears recognised and understood the dangers of the power of evil. Psychologically, the fire represents a transforming symbol.

The young man had led a sheltered life, guarded fiercely by the mother, over-protected certainly but with the best of intentions. Then suddenly one night he goes forth, and does not return until breakfast. His mother's fury knows no bounds. What occurred on the mountain? All the boy said was that he had a good time, watched the fire and saw the sun rise at dawn. What was in his mother's mind, does not take a genius to hazard a guess. But what chords were struck in the deeper realm of the boy's soul that night? He had been present at a rite which had been witnessed by untold millions of ancient peoples, to whom the sun, the mountains and the dawn represented the awesome omnipotence of Nature in its infinite majesty. Echoes of this were no doubt still reverberating through his soul as he descended the mountain, in touch with his instinctual self. Suddenly all was shattered when he was faced by the cold fury of his mother's animus.

That moment of confrontation was to be the most telling of his life. He was found wanting, unable to stand firm express himself and state his case, before this mother who had lavished all her affection, and possibly her eroticism upon him for seventeen years. This was the confrontation with the archaic image of the archetype of the mother in its negative form. Such an image would not fall short of those which have come down to us through the ages, hag, she devil, fiend, demon, or witch. Three days later the eruption began which almost cost him his life.

It is clearly connected to the events of Midsummer's Eve. One perceives a singularly destructive element in his mother's overtly solicitous approach to his well being. In the viciousness of the early morning attack, without warning on the one hand, and on the other where the surreptitious intrusion of the forbidden book is blamed upon a pretty nurse. A book which she herself had read, and then denied. The accusation against the nurse was especially wicked in that the latter had so assiduously cared for her son during his serious illness. Here is the witch, one who is possessed by a deep unconscious destructiveness, whose aim is to further the bad, or to promote evil. This deeply unconscious woman, was instrumental in plunging her son into great danger, for his life was in jeopardy for many weeks to come.

If one puts one's finger in a fire or plunges it into boiling water, the first reaction is pain, followed by its immediate reflex withdrawal in which one physically removes oneself from the source of heat. The result is a blister. When one views a patient with a multitude of blisters, tense with fluid, one is not out of order in suspecting that it is as if the being concerned has jumped into a fire, or into boiling water, he has been metaphorically burned. The fire in question, however is an inner one.

That morning on his return the young man most probably experienced a climactic volcanic eruption of rage in his soul. His rational control however together with the fear of his mother did not permit the rage to reach awareness in his consciousness. The fire however did not die down, and the emotion was not assuaged until years were to pass, and his escape was made to a new world, new in all senses. The unconscious allowed no respite until he had escaped his mother's domain, and the ambiguous thongs of her love.

The midsummer fire and the sunrise were symbolic of insight, and illumination into both his mother's personality and his own. The illness, was a rite of initiation into manhood, calling upon his heroism, by which he was enabled to overcome darkness and death. It brought into exquisite clarity the dark side of his mother of which he had only been dimly aware. Thus the illness was also a vital step in his individuation process, since only by becoming conscious can a system of personality proceed to individuate. In a retrospective review, the illness was a singular turning point.

THE RELUCTANT BRIDEGROOM

A man of middle age came to see me urgently, for he had been subjected to a most severe and overwhelming blistering disorder of the skin. The irritation and the blisters had started simultaneously seven days previously. The rash had appeared first on the head, and a few hours later on the genitals. In a matter of days it had disseminated itself symmetrically over the entire body.

When he presented himself he was in extreme discomfort, as the blisters already discharging were being replaced by new ones. He was accompanied by his wife, who was almost passive, asking no questions and giving the impression that the blatantly overt suffering of her husband was merely the reaction of a foolish cry-baby. The patient himself was close to panic, being totally overwhelmed by this distressful condition. He was apyrexial and the symmetry and the grouping of the blisters enabled the diagnosis of dermatitis herpetiformis to be made reasonably quickly at the onset, being confirmed later by histological methods. He was completely reassured as to the eventual outcome, but because of the severity of the disorder, it was decided to admit him to hospital.

In spite of concerted efforts the disease proved resistant to all forms of therapy. Unfortunately kidney complications intervened, and when these were resolved, he was again debilitated by a sudden bacterial chest infection, which was to prolong his sojourn in hospital. In all he remained for a period of seven months. On discharge, although the disorder had at last responded to therapy, it was to be almost five years before he was able to live in reasonable comfort.

During the period when difficulties were encountered in controlling the eruption, a psychological approach was adopted in order to understand the total resistance to all forms of therapy. However this proved to be a very difficult project, as profound psychic resistances became apparent.

After the initial display of panic, the man did not show any emotion again during the seven months he was under observation. As soon as he was reassured that the condition itself was not fatal he assumed like a mask, a calm demeanour. In his relationships with the nursing staff and his medical attendants he was distant, and had no social intercourse with the other patients. He had a curiously repellent habit of darting his eyes from side to side in a furtive manner, as if he was afraid although he admitted to having no fears.

He was fifty-four years of age and had been successful in his working life. By trade he was a master joiner, and had established a successful and lucrative business, and gave the impression of being quite satisfied with himself on that score. He had been married and had a family of several children. As the children left the family home, he eventually found himself alone with his wife for the first time in thirty years. Almost at once, his wife became ill, and died within a few months. The patient nursed her during the few weeks of the terminal illness, and then lived on alone in the family home, after her death. He continued with his work, and visited his married children. During the recital of his wife's illness, and his ultimate loss, he showed no sign of grief, or expressed any emotion. A few months after his wife's death he met up with a woman who was unhappily married, and living apart from her husband. In due course they decided to live together as man and wife.

The patient sold his house, and bought another in a different district. Together they set up house, entering into the life of a rather tight little community. It appeared that they were both known for their good works, and their well developed moral attitudes in the community of the new neighbourhood. Incidentally this particular locality was chosen by the wife who decided that it was eminently suitable for all their requirements. In effect, the patient forsook all his former friends and found himself greatly dis-

141

tanced from the members of his family. Eventually they were to acquire a new circle of friends and acquaintances who had not known them prior to their induction into the new neighbourhood. The man resumed his work as a joiner, and began to build up another business.

Five years later, the common law wife was divorced by her husband. The divorce became final on a Friday afternoon, and at the earliest possible hour on the following Saturday morning, the two set off quietly and got married as soon as the Registrar's office opened. They returned at once after the ceremony, did their usual weekend shopping together and celebrated at a wedding breakfast prepared by one of the wife's children. By the time that Saturday evening came to an end the even tenor of their lives had barely been ruffled by the intrusion of their wedding day.

Suddenly as night fell on the wedding night the patient began to feel uncomfortable, his skin began to itch and within a short space of time he was tearing himself to pieces. Some three or four hours after the onset of the discomfort, he remarked that blisters began to appear. He said that for a week afterwards it was as if he had entered purgatory, until he was admitted to hospital.

This history of the onset of the disorder was not easy to elicit, indeed three months were to elapse before he gave the true facts. The problem was that his wife did not wish him to divulge the secret of the recent wedding, and this fact was therefore not disclosed in the medical history. The unconscious however had no such scruples. When at last the concealment was revealed, and he did, albeit, reluctantly divulge the aforementioned history, the eruption became amenable to therapy, and was eventually controlled. Prior to his confession he had suffered from a disorder of the kidneys which in itself had proved to be intractable. After he cleared his conscience, the kidney disorder responded, but was replaced by a severe infective respiratory condition.

During the course of the discussion in which he gave me the facts concerning the début of the illness, he also told me of a dream he had had, three or four hours after he had gone to sleep somewhat fitfully on his wedding night. The dream affected him in such a way that he felt that he had awakened immediately. Furthermore when he told me of the dream, it was quite spontaneous, without prior questioning on my part. He gave it to me just after he had told me of the secret wedding. In the subsequent months before his discharge he did not admit to having had another dream. Although I got the distinct impression he found it demeaning to speak of such irrational phenomena, when he told me of his dream. I regarded it as an initial dream, and it is as follows.

Suddenly in his sleep he heard a door clang. He knew the door was huge, very heavy and by the sound he thought that it was made of metal. The clanging of the door as it shut, had reverberated for a long time, it echoed until the echoes died away and there was utter silence. Then he awoke. That was the dream, he had neither associations nor amplifications, but he was

142

certain the door was made of metal, and a joiner would of course be quite sure of the constituent materials of a door.

Psychologically this man had an extraverted attitude, his main function was sensation, and as far as his inferior function was concerned, he was not gifted with imagination. He appeared to be dissociated from his inner life completely. In spite of the wonderfully implicit dream given to him by the unconscious he was not able to make the connection between it and his outer situation, nor did he perceive any relationship between his sudden severe illness, and the time of its onset. He was a man who gave the impression of being without a soul. He was singularly unrelated, and cold.

The dream gave the prognosis of his life to be. A door did shut, and indeed from the moment that the skin disorder started he did not again recover his former good health. In the subsequent years he was to suffer from dermatitis herpetiformis for almost a decade. Just when it seemed that he was to be free of it, there arose a disabling muscular disease, which eventually invalided him completely. His muscles slowly stiffened inexorably and it appeared as if he was encased in armour. He remained remote and relatively pleasant throughout the years, adamant that he suffered no emotional difficulties, and pleased to report that he never dreamed. His wife on one occasion said, "his fault is that he is obstinate and proud". I knew she spoke the truth. Pride is one of the seven deadly sins. His pride would not allow him to admit, to the possession of one single human failing nor could he accept that another human being knew something that he did not. He was undoubtedly a good craftsman but he had identified with his vocation. One received the impression that he was incapable of taking up a new idea. It was impossible for him to envisage a reality other than the mundane world that he could see, hear, taste, smell and touch.

He had the opportunity during his first wife's illness and subsequent death to develop his feeling function, whereby it would have been possible for him to approach his inferior function of intuition. However fate decreed that he was to meet the woman who eventually became his second wife. The unconscious was against this marriage, it was a true entrapment, and when the door clanged in that fateful dream it was a turning point in his life. He had taken a wrong turn, and the inner world was lost to him. He had lost his foothold and the vital step in the individuation process which was presented to him at the time of his wife's illness, had been lost to him. Slowly over the years which were to follow his body assumed the appearance of someone slowly undergoing a process of petrification. The opportunity to transform and become conscious of his true nature was lost and with it all chances of further development.

The psychic dangers of inflation and alienation have been recognised since time immemorial, under different names, pride, conceit and arrogance. It was for this reason that taboos were provided in primitive culture to protect against just such states of inflation. Also in the Christian tradition similar protections are instituted. The seven deadly sins are all symptoms of inflation, and thus of unconsciousness, and since they are sins, confession and penance with humility were designed to guard against them. Thus the individual is kept in relationship to God, or psychologically the ego is related to the Self.

In dermatitis herpetiformis the physical pathological lesion is a subepidermal blister or split situated between the basal lamina and the dermis. The latter is the underlying nourishing supportive tissue of the former. The epidermis is therefore so to speak in danger of being adrift without anchorage, but in any event it is unsupported.

The patient was possessed of an enormous self-esteem, and by consequence his inferiorities were projected upon others. It was required of him to become conscious of his alienation, and aware of his own true reality as well as to realize his unfulfilled life especially spiritually. All this was denied him, since he could not stoop so low as to accept the grave warning contained in the humble dream which symbolized what was to be an irrevocable separation from the unconscious, the nourishment and support contained therein is vital for life as the matrix of consciousness.

It is interesting to reflect that the skin disorder exactly mirrored the psychic situation of this man. The hoped for transformation of consciousness did not take place, instead there followed a regression, with a period of stasis, before another and more severe physical disability intervened and superseded the skin disorder. If the epidermo-dermal junction in the body is representative of the physical reflection of the psychic boundary between consciousness and the unconscious, the psychic content awaiting realization can only lie at this level with the potential of possible assimilation, into ego consciousness. With the advent of the disorder of the musculature the psychic problem had become completely inaccessible to him in the deeper layers of psyche.

Eventually a crippling immobility seized his body which reflected as would a looking glass, the unexpressed affect, the deep resentments and the lonely isolation of destructive pride. Finally it was to reflect his psychic rigidity and petrification. The prophetic dream of his wedding night visualized the forthcoming entombment of body and soul.

HERPES IMPETIGINIFORMIS
THE GIRL WHO COULD NOT FACE LIFE

One evening a young woman of twenty-two years of age, noticed that her throat was sore, and her lips were swollen. She worked as a ward maid in a prestigious children's hospital, and wondered if she had caught an infection from the child patients. On awakening the next morning she discovered that her skin had begun to blister, and her body was intensely itchy. By that evening the blisters had covered the entire upper half of her body, including her face and scalp. By morning of the third day the whole body was covered with tight closely-packed blisters of the size of garden peas.

The girl decided to walk round to the casualty department of a neighbouring hospital near to where she lodged. The hospital in question was also a teaching hospital and highly regarded because of its excellence. The casualty officer suspected smallpox, and requested dermatological advices. The girl was admitted at once, the third day of her illness. Smallpox was eliminated, and the eventual diagnosis was of Impetigo Herpetiformis. The diagnosis was reached only after a great deal of reflection, upon the part, of many physicians and dermatologists called in to make the diagnosis, and with the resulting teamwork between various departmental disciplines.

I myself saw the girl for the first time on the fourth day of her illness, the morning after she was admitted. She was completely covered in blisters and her eyes were closed because the lids were swollen and replaced by purulent blistering. In addition because of gross oedema she could not raise her upper eyelids, consequently I did not see her eyes until after her death.

The latter took place four days later, and I was deeply shocked when I saw her body on the post-mortem table, with her eyes of vivid cerulean, widely opened. It appeared that they were focussed upon the forensic specialist undertaking the autopsy, with a look of what can only be described as utter disbelief.

The girl a native of Northern Europe had come to England, nine months previously in order to perfect her English.

At the time of the examination which took place when I first saw her, the blisters were already of large size, and all were either blood stained or purulent. Her mind however was crystal clear, throughout the whole short-lived illness. Because it was feared at the beginning that her disease might be contagious she was placed in strict isolation, and only the nurses who cared for her, and myself visited her regularly, apart from the senior examining physicians, who came from time to time.

The girl told me during the hours we spent together that she was an only child, her father had died when she was a baby, and she had never known him. Her mother was alive, but did not work as she suffered from a heart ailment. She had minded very much when her daughter decided to leave, and come to England. The girl however wanted to speak unaccented English, and the only way was to come and live in the country itself. She secured a job, which she liked very much, without difficulty, in a hospital. She spoke with fondness of the children with whom she was in daily contact. During the course of her duties she met a student and fell in love with him. Later she found that she was pregnant, but because the young man could not marry her, they decided together that she would have an abortion. Three months prior to the onset of her illness she had done so. After the abortion she became very sad, and felt that she had committed a terrible sin. She said that she could not shake off the feeling that she had murdered her baby.

Her constant contact with little children in the hospital heightened her sense of loss, and as the days passed she felt herself sinking deeper into a feeling of hopelessness. Each day after this confession her physical condition deteriorated rapidly, and in spite of all the medical care and expertise available, she died. I for one felt that with such a burden upon her conscience this girl could not possibly continue with her life. She told me that she was not able to forgive herself.

I met the young man who was the father of the child, just once, when it was my sad task to inform him that she had died. He was very distressed, and it was clear that he was very fond of her. After her death, her body was removed to the mortuary for an autopsy. The forensic specialist a rather well known figure in his day, and overwhelmingly autocratic, refused to perform the autopsy until a written certificate was forthcoming, verifying that the girl had not succumbed from smallpox. He had it seemed, worked in India and had seen thousands of such cases, and was deeply afraid. Eventually the certificate was produced and he proceeded. During these altercations over the body, I noticed that her bright blue eyes were open. I had the strong impression that she was listening to the arguments, an impression which I found difficult to erase, as it persisted throughout the subsequent post-mortem examination. Eventually after an exhaustive investigation it was found that no cause of death could be pin-pointed. The consensus of opinion was that cardiac arrest occurred due to a mineral/potassium/sodium imbalance.

After her death, nothing more was heard for three months, until the mortuary attendant telephoned me to state that the body had not been claimed. The mother had been told of the circumstances of her death, but had made no step to reclaim the cadaver. I enquired as to what would happen, and I was informed that her body would most probably be interred in a pauper's grave. That was the last I heard of the girl.

Sometime later, I was looking through the original records of certain cases of Impetigo Herpetiformis, which had occurred about a hundred years earlier, in the eighteen-seventies, at the lying-in hospital in Vienna. An eminent Viennese dermatologist had described twelve cases of women who had been pregnant or who were pregnant. All the women developed a severe blistering eruption described as a bullous disorder and all had succumbed from the disease within a short period of time. The connection if there is one between pregnancy and the bullous eruption has not yet been ascertained as regards the physical aspect.

I was reminded at once of this case when many years later I encountered the boy with the catastrophic mother complex, who spent Midsummer's Eve on the mountain. The distribution of the blisters and the severity both without an apparent physical cause had marked similarities. The prognosis for the boy proved in the end to be satisfactory, but for the young girl, only death awaited her.

In retrospect, I have often thought of her attitude during the time I spent with her. We were quite alone, and uninterrupted, as she was in strict isolation. She said little of her mother, who was her only remaining close relative. The impression I received was that there was considerable restraint between them, although I found the girl even in the vortex of a grave illness, to be both open and warm in her manner. The overwhelming topic of our conversation was the fact that she had committed a crime in having the abortion. She could not be pacified, and it was clear that her act weighed heavily upon her soul. The only course open to her, as she saw it, was to die, and so she did.

It was remarkable that such extraordinary fear was engendered among my senior medical colleagues when it was believed that smallpox was abroad. The fear was perfectly understandable, I also felt afraid, but at least we were all vaccinated against the disease, and some of us, many times over. I realized at the time that it was a collective fear propagated partly by the possibility of the presence of the virus itself but mostly it was a fear of the unknown. If not smallpox, what? This event took place in the sixties two decades before the world was presented with another killer-virus more insidious, more dangerous, and infinitely more invasive than the smallpox virus. Upon reflection, one can understand the gravity of the covert panic fear which has already begun to seize mankind throughout the world in the face of this new unseen threat. Behind however, is the fear of the unconscious itself.

This girl was swayed by her animus, who persuaded her to agree with her lover to dispose of the child of their union. She loved the young man, and in order to please him she opined that it was for the best. But she disregarded her deep instinctual maternalism which was far stronger than any animus opinion or outer masculine rationalism. So against this instinct she killed her child. She was undoubtedly possessed of a strong moral conscience which would not permit itself to be silenced. Throughout the subsequent period, she sank deeper into a state of melancholia. Her tie with her mother was tenuous, she could not turn to her for help, and the mother complex in its negative aspect did not provide her with inner support in her time of trial and stress. The animus succeeded in isolating her, and her illness reflected in reality this self same inner isolation. Furthermore the surrounding masculine attitude to her case was one of fear combined with bewilderment, which continued to the point of total rejection in the final phase, by her own mother who refused to accept the body. The persistently calm demeanour of the young woman in her last days belied the violence of the skin eruption. I myself have observed that the presence of blistering conditions of such appalling severity usually betokens deep unconsciousness of emotional conflicts engendering murderous rage.

Northern Europe[3] was Christianized comparatively late, round about the middle of the thirteenth century and only after considerable resistance by the adherents to the ancient pagan religions. The very oldest reports of the ancient religions are brief. However it seems that the belief of the Finno-

Ugiric people regarding the soul presents a very primitive concept. In general the disappearance of the soul was regarded as a cause of grave illness, and in such circumstances the experience of a shaman was sought, in order to retrieve the lost or errant soul and return it to the body, otherwise death would occur. The Lapps of northern Finland, whose language is also held to be Finno-Ugiric have four birth deities. They are Madderakka,[4] and her three daughters Sarakka, Jusakka, and Uksakka. Sarakka was worshipped chiefly in childbed. She also assisted the reindeer at the birth of their calves. Therefore the Lapps endeavoured not to displease her in any way. It was said that Sarakka felt the same agony as the one in childbed. Like her mother Madderakka she was believed to create the body of the infant so in fact the child was her creation. After the successful birth of a child, there was always a purification meal in honour of this goddess. Her sister Juksakka also helped to produce a child in the same way as her mother and sister, but she was also responsible for the delivery. Uksakka the third sister whose name means "door woman" was the watcher of the door, protecting all who entered or left. At childbed she received the newcomer on his arrival into the world, and guided his first steps.

The four goddesses represent a quaternity or a totality, which in a woman symbolizes the image of the Self. The concept of the total personality of psyche is a central feature of Jung's psychology. This wholeness is there to begin with but it takes time to develop. This organizing principle of the personality is an archetype which Jung calls the Self. It is the central archetype of the collective unconscious, and is the archetype of order. It is able to gather to itself to organize and to unify into an harmonious whole, all the archetypes, and their manifestations in complexes and consciousness. The Self is able to unite the personality giving it a sense of being at "one".

Upon reflection it would seem that the decision made by this young woman to abort her child was a fateful one. In reality she was a modern young woman of the Sixties, but it seemed that in her psyche there was a bonded allegiance to the old gods dynamically alive, and whom she had betrayed. Psychologically, using Jung's concept, one might be permitted to assume that she had disobeyed and gone against the Self, for which act, she forfeited her life.

PEMPHIGUS VULGARIS
THE MOTHER WHO BECAME INSANE.

A woman of twenty-eight years, pregnant with her first child had been admitted to hospital for a period of some weeks prior to the birth as there was danger of premature parturition. Two weeks before the expected arrival, it was discovered that the child had died in utero. Within twenty-four hours of receiving this news the woman began to complain of itching over the abdomen, in the region of the umbilicus. Then quite rapidly she developed an eruption consisting of blisters, the trunk in particular was seriously affected, especially in the peri-umbilical area.

A diagnosis of herpes gestationis was made, a rare non-contagious disease, occurring in pregnancy or the puerperium which is often recurrent in subsequent pregnancies. It is characterised by a subepidermal blister but current opinion believes it to be distinct from dermatitis herpetiformis. Itching is always intense, and pyrexia is common.

The woman was of the catholic faith as was her obstetrician. When the latter discovered that the foetus had died, he informed the mother at once, and told her that he would only permit the birth to proceed in the normal manner. One day later the eruption began. During the following two weeks the condition worsened, but the birth did not take place as expected. The accoucheur, reluctant to operate, decided to wait for the normal expulsion of the dead child. He waited in all ten weeks, meanwhile in the interim period the woman suffered deep dermatological distress. At last he decided to operate, and discovered that because of unforeseen pelvic abnormalities there was no possibility of a normal parturition. After the caesarian operation the woman's skin recovered almost immediately.

Some three years later she returned as an emergency, again pregnant, about a month before delivery, and again she had developed what appeared to be herpes gestationis However on this occasion it was found that the histopathology of the blisters had changed. Now it was an intraepidermal blister, whose fluid was filled with acantholytic cells. This enabled a diagnosis of pemphigus vulgaris to be made, which is a chronic blistering condition of world wide distribution. It is a disease of the middle years, and affects both sexes equally. An increased susceptibility has been confirmed in the Jewish race. The finding of auto-antibody in the sera of patients with this disorder has provided strong circumstantial evidence that there is a relationship with auto-immunity.[5] The fact of an intraepidermal blister means that it is situated in the body of the epidermis, and not at the sub-epidermal level as is observed in dermatitis herpetiformis, and herpes gestationis.

The decision was taken that the child would be delivered by means of surgical intervention at term, and this was accomplished without difficulty. The pemphigus vulgaris did not abate, but continued to increase in severity, in spite of therapeutic measures. However the most significant aspect of the post operative period was the mother's attitude towards the baby. Throughout the preceding month she had shown no anticipation, neither discussing the future birth nor the advent of her child. When the baby was presented to her after its delivery she thrust it away, and refused to feed it. When persuasive tactics were applied she admitted that she neither liked the baby nor did she want it.

Because the skin eruption was itself cause for some concern, she was retained in hospital. Some two or three weeks later she refused to hold the child which was returned to the nursery. Then she telephoned the obstetrician, and told him that voices had told her that one of the assistant male doctors had killed her baby, and hidden it in the lavatory. She then indicated that she intended to kill the doctor. This was the first intimation of a serious mental disturbance, which later involved an actual attempt upon the life of her child. The episode was described as schizophrenic and psychiatric hospitalization was required for several months. At last she was able to return to her child, when the latter was one year old. Unfortunately although chaemotherapy had provided an amelioration of the psychosis, the pemphigus vulgaris remained unchanged.

If the epidermodermal junction in the organ of the skin is equated symbolically with the border between conscious and unconscious psyche, the epidermis itself signifies inwards, from the outer corneal layer to the basal lamina the descending layers of consciousness as it approaches the level of personal unconscious. Therefore a blister or a split at the subepidermal level as has been observed represents psychically an unconscious content at the level where the potential exists for its assimilation into consciousness. With this postulation in mind, the question of the psychic meaning inherent in the intraepidermal bulla of pemphigus is raised. In this disease in both the common form and all the other varieties, the essential abnormality is disruption of the epidermal cells as a result of the loss of intercellular bridges a change known as acantholysis. It is simply a shattering or a fragmentation of the structure of the epidermis, which is no longer cohesive.

To return to the patient. During the first episode of skin disorder, which was a herpes gestationis, the blister was sited as subepidermal. Her attitude towards the situation whereby she learned of the dead baby in her womb was distant. During the subsequent period of almost three months whilst she tore herself to pieces, she displayed no real anger, either against the doctor who prolonged her suffering, or the fate which had decreed the premature death. Undoubtedly she suffered, but the lack of emotional response became evident when it was assessed against the background of the violence of the skin disease. The majority of the blisters during the episode were centred round the umbilicus.

It may be helpful to look at the symbolism of the latter, that point on the abdomen which marks the position of attachment of the umbilical cord. It centres chiefly on the omphalos a sacred, rounded conical stone in the temple of Apollo at Delphi, in Greece. This stone was believed to be both the physical and spiritual centre of the world. It was regarded as the god Apollo himself, who guarded the human race. In Celtic mythology, the menhir, had the same significance. The omphalos at Delphi was situated at the place where Apollo killed the serpent Pythia. It symbolized the vital power which dominated the blind and monstrous forces of chaos. In an individual, the psychological meaning would encompass an inner mastery over irrational fears, and unconscious affect. It is not therefore too unusual, that the blis-

150

ters, harbingers of chaotic disruption, should cluster so forcefully round the umbilical centre of this woman's body. The question which should have been posed, was why did the first child die before its birth took place?

Later when she again became pregnant, the unrecognised psychic problem of the former birth, appeared to have been resolved, in that a living child was born. This baby's birth however was to unleash a fury of demons. There had been no inkling of the severity of the underlying psychic disorder, apart from the development of the more serious skin disorder. The child was at once rejected by its malevolent mother who descended rapidly into madness, where she was to remain for the best part of a year. Had the woman been allowed to return to her home after the child's birth, there is little doubt that she would have murdered it.

The problem was a central one, in retrospect, the unconscious in its wisdom was totally against the institution of motherhood for this woman. The strange development of the relatively benign skin disease when the woman was informed that she must await the birth of the dead child was a hint of a covert emotional or psychic imbalance. The second pregnancy appeared to repeat the same pattern, but the intrusion of an infinitely more serious skin disease, although it saved the child's life eventually, was a warning of an unforeseen danger. In retrospect pemphigus vulgaris with its disruption of epidermal cell balance, reflected the fragmentation of ego consciousness and mirrored the psychosis.

TOXIC EPIDERMAL NECROLYSIS
THE CHILD WHO LIKED THE COLOUR RED.

There is a condition of the skin called toxic epidermal necrolysis, or the scalded skin syndrome, in which most of the body surface blisters, becomes red, and then the inflamed necrotic epidermis strips off in totalis. It is believed that the cause is either bacterial or drug induced. The histopathlological lesion of the latter type is a subepidermal blister.

Just such a case presented itself. A healthy little girl of four years had complained of headache and neck stiffness for which she had been given antibiotics by the family doctor. Within days she developed blisters on the trunk and what looked like a scald mark on the abdomen. A full blown toxic epidermal necrolysis developed within hours. She became very ill, and her life was threatened over a period of weeks. After six weeks of uncertainty, intensive therapy and prodigious care brought her to a full recovery. At the height of the illness, the sodden epidermis stripped away from the body, leaving raw, oozing, painful areas, similar to superficial scalds. For all the world she looked as if she had been plunged into a bath of boiling water.

After she had been in hospital for two or three weeks, it was noticed that she never spoke. Prior to the illness she had been a talkative little child,

151

very lively and energetic. The birth of a baby brother a few weeks before her illness had apparently produced a change in her personality. She had been sent away to stay with grandparents during the advent of the new child, and on return she was noticeably quieter, although she appeared to express no resentment she became wilful and demanding.

In the circumstances this would not have given rise to anxiety, but the demands centred round the colour red. She insisted that everything must be red, if new clothes were bought for her they were red likewise the clothes for her dolls, when she was admitted to hospital everything she possessed was red in colour, soap, toothpaste, toothbrush, nightgown and dressing gown.

Because of the severity of her illness this fact did not at first register. Later however it was to become quite evident that red was not just a favourite colour, but an obsession. In order to encourage her to speak again during her convalescence, her favourite sweets were presented to her. It was soon apparent that the ones she preferred were a type known as jelly babies. These are tiny moulded figures of naked children, made of sugared gelatine, and produced in a variety of colours. Furthermore a curious fact emerged. When she selected them, she carefully searched for the red ones amongst the other colours, and solemnly, silently and deliberately bit off the heads, and left the mutilated bodies. In other words she simply beheaded them, and ate the heads. It would be comparatively easy to dismiss this curious reaction and put the blame squarely upon hatred and jealousy for the new brother. Undoubtedly such an assumption would contain a strong element of truth, but not all of it. Therefore the total situation should be reviewed.

All psychologists, who have studied the development of personality will agree that the parents of a child play an extremely important rôle in this respect. Jung paid great attention to the effects of parental behaviour upon the progress and maturation of the personality of the child. During the early years of its life, its psyche is a reflection of that of its parents. Thus any disruption in their psyche is bound to be reflected in that of their child. If there appears to be a psychic problem in childhood it is essential to examine the parental psyche.

The background of the child appeared to be quite satisfactory at first, the family included the parents, the little girl and her brother. However it soon emerged, that the father of the girl was completely under the domination of his father, and the grandfather was the ruling dominant, of, not just his son's life, but of his own family and the families of his other children. His wife, the grandmother was a shadowy figure, but the daughter-in-law, the mother of the little girl was practically invisible. She was never able to visit the child alone, the husband or the grandparents always accompanied her. The grandfather took complete charge, he appeared not to permit any of the family members to air views or ask questions concerning the child's illness. He cowed those who expressed fears for her recovery.

He intruded in all discussion between the parents and the medical attendants, by questioning the therapy and the care of the little girl. He blamed the nurses for any relapse or deterioration which occurred. It transpired that this tyrannical man was a highly placed civic dignitary in his own area, and held extreme socialist views. His self-importance was increasingly engendered by intimate friendships with various members of international bodies of the same political persuasion as himself. This connection permitted him to seek advantages from locally placed governmental ministers. It became evident that he also held the female members of his family in low esteem, in particular his daughter-in-law, the mother of the sick child. It did not take too much imagination to realize the unconscious groundswell of repressed emotion in the psyche of this family. The seething resentment, and the sullen brooding anger were almost tangible and visibly perceived in the facial expression and body attitudes of its members.

The colour red played an exceptional rôle in this illness, in that the child was red, and she had a predeliction for red. There is an immense symbolism attached to this colour, which is universally considered as the fundamental symbol of the principle of life as the colour of blood and fire. It has always signified instinct and emotion. Enfolded in these ideas there is the notion of strength, power, and brilliance. Red is the secret, and sacred colour of the vital mystery hidden in the primordial oceans and the darkness. It is the colour of the heart, sexual passion, and is said to be the colour of the soul. Red in its solar aspect images the ardour and fieriness of youth, together with its beauty. The red paint used by young African women, and both the young men and women of some North American Indian tribes is supposed to stimulate and arouse sexual desire. In Russia, China and Japan it has always been associated with popular festivals, especially those of Springtime, birth and marriage. It is a colour of renewal, as was apparent when this colour was adopted by the revolutionaries during the 1917 Russian revolution. It represented the blood lost, the anger of the Bolshevics, and the new era for the revolutionary powers of the masses. Since then red has become synonymous with Communism, later it was to symbolize the whole of red China, as well as the surrogate Marxist nations.

In ancient Celtic lore, red was the colour of the warrior representing a very old tradition. Dagda the druid god was Ruadh Rofhessa 'a red of the great science'. The druids were often called red druids, because they were at once, warriors, and also priests to the warriors.[6]

The fire was central to the alchemical opus, the athanor was never allowed to go out. It signified the central fire of the work, the libido or psychic energy required to complete the opus. It was sometime called the red work, from which issued the transformed. One of the alchemical stages was the rubedo. Jung[7] in quoting from 'Rhasis' says "The stone first an old man, in the end a youth, because the albedo comes at the beginning and the rubedo at the end".

In alchemy the fire purifies, but it also melts the opposites into a unity.

In describing the coming of illumination in the alchemical process Jung[8] has this to say:

> "The situation is now gradually illuminated as is a dark night by the rising moon. The illumination comes to a certain extent from the unconscious, since it is mainly dreams that put us on the track of enlightenment. This dawning light corresponds to the albedo the moonlight which in the opinion of some alchemists heralds the rising sun. The growing redness (rubedo) which now follows, denotes an increase of warmth and light, coming from the sun, consciousness. This corresponds to the increasing participation of consciousness which now begins to react emotionally to the contents produced by the unconscious. At first the process of integration is a "fiery" conflict but gradually it leads over to a "melting" or synthesis of the opposites. The alchemists termed this the rubedo in which the marriage of the sun man and the white woman Sol and Luna is consummated. Although the opposites flee from one another they nevertheless strive for balance since a state of conflict is too inimical to life to be endured indefinitely. They do this by wearing each other out: the one eats the other, like the two dragons or the other ravenous beasts of alchemical symbolism".

Jung's eloquent words describing the rubedo have been quoted in full, in order to portray the infinitely mysterious process of resolution of the conflict of the opposites.

In all these cases described where a severe blistering eruption suddenly entered into a life, it was the physical manifestation of a severe inner psychic conflict. With the case of the first young man, it was an unresolved mother complex, the illness afforded him the opportunity to realize the duality of the archetype. His period of suffering in hospital constituted the rubedo. The old masculine attitude of submission to the feminine was transformed into that of a liberated male. The Nordic girl lost her life, the rubedo did not achieve an earthly transformation, wholeness was only possible in death. The bridegroom did not achieve an increase in consciousness, au contraire, he regressed, and for him the result was a death in life.

With this child, she was the victim, the problem lay elsewhere. She was the reflector of a maelstrom of fury in the family. The mother of the little girl was subjected to vile tyranny at the hands of the aged grandfather. She was supported neither by her fearful husband, nor the timid grandmother. Furthermore she was quite unable to express herself against the overwhelming burden of her own inner rage, and the outer despotic exercise of power. Interestingly enough the appearance of the child was exactly as if she had been burned or scalded, just as if she had been in outer contact with extreme heat. The disease process of the child was in fact or so it seemed, a portrayal of a deeply unconscious and unresolved familial conflict. The unconscious instinctual rebellion on the part of the mother against the grandfather's Marxist ethos was reflected in the colour of the child's damaged skin, its choice of possessions, and the chosen sweets. A jelly baby is an homunculus, a tiny man or a dwarf. In alchemical union, an embryo was produced, whose equivalents were the lapis or an homunculus.

One may be permitted to conjecture that the whole disease process was an exteriorised image of the unconscious endeavouring to portray the conflict and produce a solution. The ingestion of the heads of the homunculi appears then as an attempt to assimilate consciousness of the situation, the head serving as the receptacle of consciousness. As a symbol, the homunculus would represent union of both conscious and unconscious. Certainly in the family situation there was no evidence of heightened consciousness, nor any evidence of transformation. However the child was transformed, she recovered completely from the severe illness, her speech was regained, and before her return to her home she began to draw. Her favourite red pencil was used to depict a smiling lady who was she said, her mother. It was an image of that lady which I had not had, nor did I have the opportunity to verify. Perhaps it was simply the observer who was destined to witness and try to understand the evolution of this miraculous event in a child's life.

REFERENCES

1 Frazer, J. G., Manhardt, W., The Golden Bough, Chapter LXIII.
2 Frazer, J. G., Westermenck, E., The Golden Bough, Chapter LXIII.
3 Mythology of all Races, Vol. IV Chapter I.
4 Ibid., Vol. IV p. 253.
5 Rook, A., Wilkinson, D. S., Ebling, F. J. G., Textbook of Dermatology, 3rd Edition. Vol. 2, p. 1453, Blackwell Publications.
6 Windisch, Ernst, Irische Text, 5 vols., Leipzig, 1880–1905, Passim. Ogam Tradition Celtique Rennes, 1948, 12. 452–458.
7 Jung, C. G., Collected Works, Vol. 14, para 7 n. 34 "Opusulum Autoris ignoti" Art aurif I, p. 390, Routledge & Kegan Paul, London.
8 Jung, C. G., Collected Works, Vol. 14, para 307, Routledge & Kegan Paul, London.

10

ERYTHRODERMA

One of the most severe dermatological disorders is a condition called Erythroderma which simply means red skin. It can intervene at any stage of a chronic dermatosis. Included in this group are those cases of reactions due to drug sensitisation, chronic eczema, psoriasis, cases due to blood dyscrasias, or cancerous change. When it arises, it appears as if the body can no longer hold in check, an hithertofore chronic process, which begins to flare uncontrollably, like wildfire. It is a chaos of the skin, and is always a catastrophe. Many who develop this condition succumb, either earlier or later. For those who survive, usually years pass before the skin again achieves a state of equilibrium. The French give the singularly apt name of L'Homme Rouge' to the condition because of the colour of the skin. The latter is a violent fiery glowing red, which can range from a deep magenta colour, to a coppery bronze. Constant scaling is a serious feature, which leads to a marked protein depletion.

In the many patients with erythroderma, whom I have encountered over the years, there have been few occasions to undertake more than a relatively superficial psychic assessment. This is due to the grave nature of the disease process itself which is not conducive for more serious study. Except for two sufferers from the malady who were inmates of psychiatric institutions, the others whom I have treated showed no evidence of overt psychic derangement. However in spite of this I have been forced in time, to regard erythroderma as a 'psychosis' of the skin. The long periods of incapacity spent in hospitals or clinics appear to be necessary not just for the cure of the skin, but also to achieve a psychic adjustment in the individual concerned. Thereby the psychic equilibrium itself is protected whilst the organ of the skin acts as a buffer in order to carry the 'chaotic' state.

'LA FEMME ROUGE'

A married woman in her twenties complained of a sore throat, which resulted from a bacterial infection. Eventually a tonsillar abscess or quinsy developed. She was given chaemotherapy, but a severe hypersensitivity to the particular drug intervened and it became necessary to hospitalise her. The drug allergy did not subside, as was expected, instead over some weeks she developed erythroderma. She remained in hospital for a year but two years were to elapse before her skin achieved a stable state. During the recovery she suffered renal complications which almost took her life.

Although this woman was very ill, and there was real danger that she might not survive, her attitude was very difficult. She was opinionated to a degree, autocratic, and disagreeable. She professed herself anxious for recovery, but her general demeanour belied it. She questioned every aspect of her therapy and usually rejected it. There was a refusal of all foods and medicaments prescribed which she usually considered to be useless or dangerous. Her resistances led to a serious deterioration in her condition. Finally the nursing staff found her so objectionable they refused to nurse her.

It was at this juncture that the decision was made to inform her in the strongest terms of the exact nature of her illness and indicate the precarious prognosis. This approach, unusual to say the least was undertaken with the idea to shock her opinionated and fractious animus. Fortunately it succeeded. Overnight, after this fright she became obedient, and shortly her behaviour proved to be exemplary. This change of attitude on her part was the turning point of the illness. Many setbacks were still to occur but her increased consciousness saved her, from herself. She had been on a collision course to death.

This young woman had been the only child of her parents' marriage. When she was three years old, her father had died. A year or so later the mother remarried and the family went abroad, to live. At the tender age of seven years, the little girl was sent to boarding school in the country of her birth, she rarely saw her parents, being cared for by guardians.

The woman explained that she disliked her stepfather and felt uncertain about her mother, receiving the impression that she had not been wanted. I did not disagree with her assumption. At school she was bright and intelligent and at twenty-two she launched herself into the world of computer technology after leaving the university. A year later she married a man in the same field. There were no children of the marriage, which was apparently satisfactory.

It was noted during the illness that the husband came infrequently, made no enquiries as to her welfare, and never stayed very long. Excuses were made on his behalf to account for his lapses, and were usually centred round his busy life.

When her recovery was assured she was allowed to go home, with the proviso that she returned for regular tests, on account of her continued medication. Her first appointment was not kept, and she was not seen again for almost a third of a year.

When she returned eventually, she gave the following report. Since her husband was not able to collect her, she went home alone. As she entered the kitchen she noticed a cactus pot plant on the kitchen table. Propped against it was a letter from her husband which explained that the plant was a good-bye present. In the letter he made it clear that he had left her for someone else, adding that he hoped she would consider divorce. There was not a word of welcome, comfort or hope. This was the greeting after a year of grave illness, during which time her life had been in jeopardy.

Such a letter is a death blow. At first she thought of suicide, but was able to control herself sufficiently to telephone a relative in North America. Within a day or so she found herself cared for by a kindly woman who left her in peace to recover physically, and repair the deep psychic wound.

The woman said that since it was winter time she walked daily in the snow to regain her strength and when she could not do so she gazed at the ice-bound window panes, where ice crystals formed and reformed themselves into snow flower shapes.

When she returned home, she agreed to divorce her husband, and she decided to leave the masculine world of technocracy. She eventually became a master craftsman-jeweller working with gold and precious stones. The idea seemingly came to her, as she observed the snow flower patterns in the winter.

In retrospect the woman's illness was a transformation of her entire personality. It began with an abscess of the tonsils a quinsy which is an obstruction to the act of swallowing. Although the marriage appeared to be satisfactory one might surmise that psychically there was an unconscious problem which could not be swallowed. However she became allergic to the proposed cure, of antibiotic therapy. On admission she resisted everything. It was clear that there was an unconscious wish to die, a state which is often seen when life becomes quite intolerable for one reason or the other. She professed her anxiety to live, but her acts did not support her statements.

She had a serious shadow problem. Jung gave the name of shadow to the archetype which represents one's own gender, and influences those relationships with others of one's own sex. The shadow contains more of man's basic animal nature than the other archetypes, therefore in the civilizing process this nature is restrained by developing a strong persona which acts against the shadow's power. However in suppressing the shadow, creative impulses, insights, spontaneity and strong emotions are banished. Thereby the individual is cut off from the irreplaceable wisdom of instinctual nature.

When she entered the computer world, in order to survive, this intelligent woman had to conform to a specific image. She became hard working, diligent, dependable and responsible. This was her persona. In Jung's psychology the persona archetype enables one to present a character which is not necessarily one's own. It is a mask. Unfortunately she identified with it and by so doing became inflated, and this caused an increase in unconsciousness. In fact she was no longer a woman. She had treated her womanly self for a long time with the same brutal coldness which she realized and at last encountered in her husband's barbarism.

In the hospital she was given feminine support throughout the year, the care and attention provided by the nursing staff was accompanied by real feeling. Probably this was the first time she had been the recipient in her life. Undoubtedly it enabled her to support herself when she received her husband's letter.

The cactus plant is quite significant. Being a succulent it is able to retain moisture, and thus can survive for years without water, and can withstand severe drought. It is prickly to ward off predators, and protect itself. Many years sometimes pass before a cactus blooms, but often when it does it produces a flower of exquisite even unearthly beauty.

The husband's choice of present probably depended on the easy availability and cheapness of such a plant. However as an unconscious choice representative of feeling, the cactus indicated superbly the inaccessible nature of his wife's inferior function, and also his own.

The snowscape in North America indubitably reflected the inner coldness, and desolation of the woman herself. The continual observation of the snow flowers, was in fact the formation and reformation of mandalas. She was witnessing unconsciously her own inner psychic transformation. It was this fascinating observation which led her to work eventually with gold and jewels, the earth's treasures, which symbolize treasures of the unconscious.

She had permitted conscious ego to play too dominant a rôle in her personality, thereby neglecting to individuate and express the shadow side of her nature, until the illness. The latter gave her a year to regain her wholeness.

The recovery from the grave malady of erythroderma 'L'Homme Rouge' or as in her case 'La Femme Rouge' represented the symbolic passage through the rubedo of the alchemical process. The slow physical transformation took place over a period of two years. However at the same time a profound psychic transformation was also occurring. This however could only be observed after her recovery and in retrospect. At last its stability and its beauty could be seen in her physical transformation together with the outer transformation of her life.

11

CONNECTIVE TISSUE DISEASES
Lupus Erythematosus

Lupus Erythematosus is a skin disease which may be of a localised or generalised form. It is usually classed as a connective tissue disease. This term has replaced the older "collagen disease". A description which is in fact unacceptable because the collagen appears not to be at fault. Of late other terms are used on account of the increasing emphasis on immunological abnormalities. This has brought the names of "auto-immune diseases" and "immunological" disease to these conditions. In most skin circles, the term connective tissue disorder is still current.

(1) LOCALISED LUPUS ERYTHEMATOSUS

A middle aged married woman presented with an area of baldness on the top of her head. It looked exactly like the tonsure of a monk or a priest. The hairless skin was pink, shiny smooth and thin, and covered the whole vertical area of the scalp. To cover it she wore a partial wig, which she called a transformation. The advancing edge of the bald area was raised, revealing active disease.

She explained that she had seen both specialists and doctors in the twenty-seven years since the condition first appeared, at the age of twenty. At first she thought that she had burned her scalp or injured it in some way, but the bald area gradually increased as the years passed. A diagnosis of discoid lupus erythematosus was made, which is the localised chronic form of a connective tissue disorder. It had been treated with all the pertinent and available medicaments including courses of anti-malarial drugs, extending over

160

long periods of time. However nothing had stopped the slow, insidious and inexorable progress of the disease process, and the area of advancing baldness continued. After undertaking her case it was eventually realized that the condition was intractable without any evidence of favourable progress.

One day she told of a dream, which had upset her profoundly, in which her doctor had pushed a mercurial thermometer right down into her throat, and was choking her to death. She woke up in great distress and found that her mouth was full of blood. The doctor, whom she liked, was a middle aged man, he had been her practitioner for many years, and he was very competent. She said that she thought he was trying to take her temperature, and did not seem to know that he was killing her. It puzzled me as to why the unconscious would portray him in such a light. It appeared that the dream depicted a frantic effort to establish the presence of fever, on the doctor's part. I began to wonder that perhaps a different approach to her problem was required. It was then that I decided to investigate her psyche. Until that time I had not thought consciously of a psychic background to the connective tissue disorders. She produced few dreams, and those which followed were at long intervals apart. The decision was made to undertake a word association experiment, which Jung developed in the early years of this century, and she agreed to it.

During the test she faltered on the stimulus word "marriage" and could not recall the former lapse in the re-run of the test. These results were both highly interesting and totally unexpected, as she had led me to believe that her marriage was ideal. In fact the word association experiment had touched upon the very heart of her emotional problem which, it came to light later, had co-existed with the baldness for almost thirty years. The marriage problem was a secret, known only to herself. In a strange way the baldness, concealed by the transformation hair piece was a reflection of the inner situation. The word association test proved invaluable in this case. Indeed it is a tool of immense potential in those cases where dissociation is the pertinent problem.

The woman with the unfaithful husband

After the word association experiment and during the course of several months, the story which unfolded revealed that she had married at the age of twenty, and had conceived her only child during the honeymoon. Some time later, during the pregnancy, she discovered that her husband was unfaithful. She was very distressed and went into a depression which lasted several months. It was during this period, just after the birth of her child that she became aware of the advancing bald patch on the crown of her head. She explained that she would have left her husband, but for the sake of the unborn child she stayed with him. Apparently he decided to give up the woman with whom he had had a relationship for some time, prior to

161

the marriage. However during the course of the marriage itself the question of the husband's repeated infidelities was to surface again from time to time. When she was asked why she continued to support the situation she could give no reason. She replied "I just stay".

She had cared for the home, brought up her child, and secured a good job for herself, and continued as if the marriage was satisfactory. Indeed on one level she had persuaded herself that it was "ideal"; and she believed it. Furthermore she had never discussed the problem with anyone. During the three decades of her marriage, she had suffered several bouts of depression. Later it was discovered that these all correlated with her husband's infidelities and were followed by an exacerbation of her scalp condition.

This pleasant woman was both kind and intelligent, her superior function was extraverted feeling, with thinking as her inferior function. In order to continue with the marriage she pushed away all thoughts related to the transgressions of her husband. She refused to permit them to shatter the serenity of her life. But the thoughts did not vanish, they were propelled into the unconscious, and so instead of suffering the conflict consciously she suffered long lonely bouts of depression.

After she had been treated for a year, she had a short series of dreams, of which three had the same motif. In each she was aboard a sailing ship heading for the New World. Although she knew that she was a passenger, she was uncomfortably aware that she was also the captive of an unknown man. In the first dream she was imprisoned below decks, and her gaoler was a brutish tyrant. In the second dream the unknown man was a slave master, the owner of several slaves; and in the third dream he was a sinister ship's captain. She described the latter as cold and brutal, and she added that in the dream she was mortally afraid of him.

The dreams clearly demonstrated the nature of the animus. She was undoubtedly bound for the new world, in that she had entered the territory of the unconscious realm by way of her analysis. She was also in fact a passenger, as she allowed herself to be carried in life, and she was most certainly a captive in her total life situation. She was tyrannised by the coldly brutal, and indeed sadistic animus. The animus as the masculine unconscious of woman, is the unknown inner masculine being, of which she is usually completely unaware. He is perceived in dreams, and by projection is encountered in the outer world. In the case of this woman he was portrayed as being a man in charge, as the sea captain, and also as both slave and taskmaster and gaoler. As her inner guide and psychopompos he had led her into a marriage where she was to become a prisoner and confined to captivity for almost three decades. When questioned about the marriage, the animus spoke, and the woman made statements such as "she ought to stay", "she should fulfil her duties as a wife", "she must accept her husband's nature", (and also his profligacy.) It was as if she mentally genuflected and submitted in prostration. It seemed that she was hypnotised by her husband, as would be a rabbit before a cobra. On closer inspection, a different picture emerged. Although it was certainly true that she feared her husband the cause of her real terror lay within. Slowly she came to accept the brutal tyranny of the negative thoughts of her animus as he entered from the unconscious through the open door of her inferior thinking function. The hideous nature of such thoughts was intolerable in her bovine Christian consciousness and not to be accepted. Thus they were despatched, but not lost. They formed the nucleus of what might be described as an infidelity complex, which in time became the instigator of long periods of black depression.

When eventually, and with immense difficulties she began to perceive the nature of her unconscious masculine self, she found that depression was no longer such a burden for her. It was about this time, a year after the captive dreams, that the advancing edge of the discoid lupus erythematosus underwent a change. Naturally the baldness did not recover, but the progress of the disease was halted. She was then able to deal, very slowly, with the problem of her husband's infidelity.

Her appearance was suggestive of a scalping. Flaying and scalping are closely connected, and since the former signifies a transformation from a worse state to a better, as has been seen, this also holds good for scalping. Thus ideas of renewal and rebirth, are connected with it. Ancient Mexico with its old religious rites was renowned for the flaying, scalping and decapitation ceremonies. Shaving of the head has long been associated with consecration, which signifies a spiritual initiation or transformation. The meaning of the tonsure is enfolded in these ideas. As Jung[1] explains "the 'symptom' of the transformation goes back to the old idea that the transformed one becomes like a new born babe . . . with a hairless head".

In submitting to the tyranny of the animus, the patient had set her face against her instinctual feminine nature and had come to treat herself in the same denigrating and churlish manner as did her husband over the years, in the outer reality world. In the only way possible the unconscious throughout the years had urged for a spiritual transformation, a much needed change of attitude. Through the medium of the body an image was presented to her. The somatic tonsorial baldness became the perfect reflection of the required psychic change. This is an example of how the unconscious thinks. Interestingly enough, in order to cover the "shame" of the denuded area, she bought herself a hair piece or transformation as she described it. What was required was a transformation by way of a consecration to the Self, the archetype of wholeness.

The disease discoid lupus erythematosus is characterized histopathologically by two features. A degeneration of the living basal cell layer of the epidermis, and also a fibrinoid change of the connective tissue immediately below it. This petrifying process of the skin was mirrored exactly by the obduracy of the animus in the brutal impact he made against her feminine nature.

(2) GENERALISED LUPUS ERYTHEMATOSUS
THE GIRL WHO LOVED HER DOG

A young girl of 17 years came to see me with a skin disease affecting her face, and a type of rheumatism affecting the small joints. Eventually the diagnosis of generalised lupus erythematosus was made.

She was undoubtedly ill, but her manner was disagreeable, and she was both sullen and moody. She had an intense redness of the face which looked like a fiery blush, but was not of a temporary nature. It had the distinct pattern of a butterfly, which is a classical sign of lupus erythematosus, with a red nose, forehead and cheeks. She came with her mother, who seemed to be in a hurry to go elsewhere. The mother was decidedly off-hand about her daughter's illness. The rheumatoid specialists who had been treating her had instituted high doses of steroids, therefore it was decided that I should see her regularly on a monthly basis, to observe the progress of the skin condition. I decided quite early on that she should come alone, without the mother (much to the latter's relief). From the dermatological point of view the butterfly rash was the most important sign.

Symbolism of the Blush

The blush is a strange phenomenon for which the conscious self feels no responsibility and which it cannot control. The ancient Romans had a curious custom, whereby if someone blushed, he at once rubbed his forehead. It was believed at that time that the "genius" resided in the head, and therefore by touching the forehead, deference was made to him, it was an act of propitiation. According to Onians,[2] the word genius was in origin the Roman analogue of the word 'psyche', the life spirit in procreation, dissociated from and external to the conscious self. The latter was believed to reside in the centre of the chest. The genius was thought to assume the form of a snake, as did the psyche.

In those days the Romans held the view that the head itself was the source of the seed, and thus concerned in procreation. This perhaps explains the associations of "the word genius, with gigno, genus and lecto genialis".[3] The forehead particularly was sacred to the genius, which was believed to be that part of man which survived his death, as did the psyche of the Greeks. The departed spirit of the dead person was sometimes referred to as his genius. In life however it was honoured as a god, a status naturally associated with immortality.

The head is primarily affected by honour, dishonour, and shame. One raises one's head high in an honourable act, or bows one's head in disgrace or shame. Thus one can easily understand the need to propitiate the god. Interestingly enough the Romans described the blush as a fire, a particularly apt description, accompanied as it is by a subjective burning sensation

164

and feelings of warmth. The latter results from an actual rise in skin temperature, being thus a psychosomatic reaction. Since shame as well as rage is always accompanied by redness and burning of the head, in Roman thought the blush came to be associated with the emotion of shame. Ordinary rage was thought to be concerned with the conscious self, but furious rage was a different entity. In the latter, the face was reddened, the face and head swollen, the eyes bulged and the hair stood on end. In such cases it was believed that the life soul was dangerously involved, and the individual was thought to be going out of his mind.

A condition of the skin, by the pretty name of Acne Rosacea, is signified by a marked redness of the face and the eyes, with swelling of the tissues. When analysed, often a monumental anger is exposed, usually concealed for many years, in an ongoing conflict situation. Such a man attended for therapy, he had married a shrew, and a rich one at that. He never contradicted her, or expressed himself in any way, but over the years this non-drinking man developed a face that was of a fiery red, with permanently protruding eyes and swollen tissues. He had the appearance of one who was about to burst into a maniacal rage, yet he was softly spoken, and gentle in manner. One afternoon, I brought up the subject of his wife, a strange look passed over his face, and then he looked at his watch, and said that it was time for him to leave. I had mentioned the tender spot in his psyche, the cause of a deep unconscious and terrible rage, and perhaps the real cause of it was his deep sense of shame for his failure as a man to contradict his wife.

With these ideas concerning the blush the case of the young woman is again considered. As I got to know her better she remained sullen, and disinclined to discuss her illness, but she did attend regularly and she did wait patiently through long and tedious clinics. After about three months, when her condition slowly deteriorated, I asked her one day how the condition had begun. She answered, that it had just started.

Then I asked her when it had started. This is, I have found the most important question that can be asked about an illness.

The answer always holds the vital key. She looked directly at me, and said "July 16, 19..". I was taken totally by surprise, she gave me the exact date, month and year. The date itself was six months previous to the date of the actual consultation, when I asked her the question. I then asked her how she had remembered. She told me that, she was looking after the dog, because her parents had gone on holiday.

It transpired that the girl, sixteen years old at the time, had been left alone in the house, which was quite large, except for the dog. I asked her if she had wanted to accompany them, but she said that she did not, she wanted to look after the dog. It became obvious that the dog was of course, infinitely more important in her life than were either of her parents. The question which had been asked proved to be a turning point in her life.

165

Symbolism of the Dog

The symbolism of the dog is far too vast to be dealt with other than in a cursory way. The dog symbolizes relatedness. It is the companion of Asklepios the god of doctors, and is a psychopompos which leads to the other world. It has a good nose representing the function of intuition, and can sniff out possibilities for good as well as evil. The dog is also associated with death. The card, numbered eighteen of the Tarot, depicts two dogs, howling at the full moon in front of a gate. This card is sometimes called the Hecate, after the death goddess whose companions were dogs. Her gates were guarded by Cerebeus, the three headed, 'Spirit of the pit'. The hounds of the goddess Hel, were lunar wolf dogs, whose leader was Managarm (Moon Dog). Dogs were the natural companions of the huntress, but also the housewife in their capacity as guards.

To return to the young woman. A few weeks after the above conversation, I found that we had established a good relationship to each other. She began to smile, and became quite friendly. One day as I was looking back through her case report, I saw on one page a small entry, 'termination of pregnancy'. It was handwritten by an obstetrician with a comment that it was at the instigation of the mother.

This information which had been "forgotten" by the mother, the girl, and the rheumatologist was very interesting. It had taken place about a year earlier. I asked the girl when the baby would have been born, and without a trace of hesitation, she answered (July 16, 19..) the date that the systemic lupus erythematosus had started, six months after the abortion.

The girl said that she was very upset about the abortion, she loved the boy very much, and wanted to have the baby. Her mother was very angry, and refused to allow her to have it. She had said they were both too young to marry, the girl said that she cried for a week, then the family doctor and her mother insisted that a psychiatrist was called in. The latter had also fallen in with the mother's view, and the consensus of opinion was that they all considered that abortion would be the best solution. Sometimes, owing to the immaturity of the girl abortion is the best solution, but in this case it clearly was not. The incredible "coincidence" of the expected birth and the development of the disease, in which the primary lesion is fibrinoid necrosis, or death of the flexibility of tissue, was a synchronistic event.

This girl had been forced to go against her instincts, and her innate feminine nature had been murdered, along with the unborn child. By staying at home, to care for her dearly loved dog, that significant week, when she expected to have become a mother, was crucial in her life. The date of the unexpected birth was fixed in her mind.

When a child is conceived the body of a woman is programmed for a monumental change, in which the life of the new child-to-be takes paramount place. When suddenly and before naturally ordained, the programme

166

is halted in full expansion, one can only wonder at the disruption of those bodily changes which must ensue. Such an abortion, against the instincts of the woman herself is an act against Nature. In this instance the girl desired the child.

The young woman was eminently normal and intelligent, and possessed of a good instinct. She grasped the situation at once. Over a long period we discussed the young man who stayed with her for two years, in spite of her mother's disapproval. In the end, however he left her, since the mother refused their marriage.

With regard to the parents, both were rational, sure of themselves, not given to self-doubt, and unfeeling in their attitude to their daughter. The mother was distinctly objectionable without warmth, and she brought with her the cold chill of evil.

After three years of therapy this young woman made a good recovery. The butterfly rash began to clear as soon as the abortion was 'aired'. Some seven or eight years later she met another man, married him and became the proud and excellent mother of twins. She had no further trouble, and ten years later was reported to be fit and well.

It seemed to me that the rash signalled the dishonourable way her inner iuno or genius had been treated. She had gone against the Self. The fear, and the abject terror which she experienced in the unconscious was reflected in the stiffened and petrified limbs, particularly the hands and feet. This girl was undoubtedly the victim of her mother's evil nature. The baby which was killed was her own grandchild, offspring of her only daughter. She was possessed by a ferocious animus who brooked no interference, as she overwhelmed her daughter, subjugated her husband and persuaded three physicians to do her bidding. Her actions revealed a singular unrelatedness and absence of Eros. The disease which beset her daughter produced a generalised petrification, and stiffening of the body. Just such a condition which befell those who saw the Medusa. Indeed here was a mother complex in its most destructive and negative aspect.

The girl however had a good 'dog' that is a sound instinct, relatedness, and a healthy intuition. She was able with feminine support to realize that she had unwillingly, and unwittingly, been the pawn forced to act against the interest of the life force. This case demonstrates the way in which Nature avenges herself when wronged. It also reveals that extreme circumspection should be exercised when medical decisions of such importance, as in this girls case, are undertaken.

(3) MORPHOEA OR SCLERODERMA

This is a rare condition which may be localised or generalised. It is of unknown cause, and is characterized by sclerosis of the skin, in which the dermis is thickened, and the elastic tissue reduced. In the localised form there are generally a single plaque, guttate or linear lesions whereas in the generalised form, vast areas of the body are affected, involving the trunk, breasts, abdomen and thighs. Sometimes a generalised form may develop from an extension of the localised form. Localised morphoea tends to undergo spontaneous resolution over the years, sometimes over periods as long as quarter of a century. New lesions however do tend to reappear. The generalised form also tends to improve, but the length of the disease often extends over decades. The danger to the patient is immobility due to sclerotic changes and contractures in the limbs. In those patients where the whole body is affected, the appearance is suggestive of armour plating.

The Swimmer

A young girl of thirteen years was referred because of a sudden stiffening of the buttocks, the lower trunk posteriorly and the upper thighs. The condition had been present for some weeks, her mobility was impeded, and her walking was severely affected. The real reason for the referral however was because the girl could no longer swim. This in fact was the paramount problem. Both the girl's mother and the physician in charge were concerned about this fact, not, surprisingly, that the girl was rapidly becoming immobile. A diagnosis of generalised morphoea was made.

The young girl explained that the trouble had started one afternoon quite suddenly. Before that day she had been perfectly alright, she believed. She had gone with friends for a picnic in the woods and whilst sitting on a stone wall at the boundary of the woods, she suddenly felt her buttocks go cold and stiff. When she got home the sensation persisted. It is difficult to be certain as to whether the condition did actually start then or not, but the girl believed it did. Moreover the mother of the girl noticed the unusually coloured areas on the buttocks and thighs the next day when she was preparing to go swimming.

The anamnesis is as follows. The girl was an only child, the parents were divorced when she was six years old, and she had been brought up, apparently in an exemplary fashion by the mother. The father had remarried after the divorce but the girl saw him several times a year, and was fond of him. Swimming had become very important in her life. She swam well and had received a great many medals and decorations. She trained for international events, and there was a possibility that she might enter major international games in due course, when she was of age. In order to achieve this she had to practice swimming for two or three hours before she started school, and for two or three hours when she finished school every day. She also swam on Sunday mornings. The girl had no recreation, her mother did not allow her to go out with her friends, and she had no time for hobbies. She was not allowed to indulge herself in any way. Her life centred solely round swimming. She professed strongly that she liked it.

With the onset of her illness the prognosis depended in the early stages upon therapy and adequate rest for the child. Surprisingly the mother became very angry and refused to accept both the diagnosis, and the suggestion that swimming should be abandoned for the time being. She refused to accept all advices, and brought a man friend to support her, and add weight to her arguments. The mother was adamant that the girl should continue to train in spite of the weakness of the back and lower limbs. She opined that the body would be strengthened with the exercise entailed in the daily practice. Be it, remembered, the girl could barely walk, because of the thickening and swelling of the tissues of the lower half of the body.

Fortunately after weeks of argumentation during which the girl's condition deteriorated, a note of wisdom came by way of the girl's father, who delivered the last word by forbidding the child to continue the training. Here was a positive, supportive father, who discerned the problem quite clearly, and acted with alacrity. One may compare his reaction, with that of the weak father in the previous case, who allowed the mother to overwhelm the daughter.

It seemed important to ask what the girl had been doing when she sat upon the stone wall. She said that it was a lovely sunny day, and she was in the company of friends. She thought how agreeable it was to have nothing to do, but listen to her friends, and talk to them.

This girl had been isolated from the companionship of her peers by the ambition of her mother. She had been coerced into the competitive world of sport, and forced to conform to her mother's iron will. No recognition was permitted of the child's feelings, her individual wishes, or even her dislikes. She was the puppet of the mother – an extension of her will. Apparently, in later years, it was revealed that the mother had wanted as a girl, to be a swimming champion. Unfortunately her physical strength was limited, as she had not the muscular power required for sustained swimming. Her daughter possessed this muscular strength, and so the mother was able to live the sporting life, vicariously through that of her child.

Scleroderma or morphoea produces an iron hard skin. The aim of therapy is to soften it, and restore mobility. A characteristic feature of the condition is a mask-like facies. The face becomes smooth, rigid and stiff. Consequently the smile is slow to develop, and persists a long time before it fades away. In cases with this condition, often only the eyes are quick, alert and mobile. This appearance often resembles that of an animal. Emotion is rarely revealed on such a face, so affected, and it is difficult therefore to read the expression. In the case of this girl, the face was completely normal, but singularly, the buttocks presented a similar picture of complete rigidity. They had the appearance of a death mask.

169

Symbolism of the Mask

A mask is equivalent to a chrysalis. In ancient Italian practice, a mask or likeness of the head was often hung up to secure fertility, which is the natural work of the genius of the procreative spirit. Such an oscillum was also hung up for the departed spirit, when a man died by hanging. A copy of the head sometimes was placed in the grave at a normal funeral, for the same reason. Onians[4] believes that perhaps this is the reason why the words 'larva' which means ghost, and mask is used. The medieval Latin word 'masca' means goblin and also mask. The word mask occurs in many non-European languages and might be traced to the Sumerian word 'maskim' which has the meaning of spirits or ancestral ghosts a similar meaning to the Latin word larva. The Sufi magicians were said to be 'maskhara' or revealers. The word 'masca' remained one of the church's official names for witch.

To put on a mask is to become another, it is to undergo a metamorphosis by which one is transformed, whilst yet remaining the same. The mask as the agent of transformation is invested with a mysterious essence in which are enfolded ideas of both concealment and revelation, as well as death, and continued life. A theatre actor dons a mask and plays a part, but as the new character is created the actor, as a man, remains the same. His life continues throughout the play, as the actor; but the character portrayed is forever born anew, as the personality of the actor disappears behind the mask, at the start of each performance and is reborn anew at the end.

From earliest times, the mask has held pride of place in ancient religions, since it was believed that deity resided in the sacred mask. Thus the wearer of such was possessed by the spirit of the god, and he or she became the god or goddess. Or if a witch doctor of a primitive tribe donned the mask of an animal, he was not pretending that he was the animal, he had a psychic identity with the creature. The mask has always played a vast and varied rôle in primitive societies, particularly in the rites of initiation, agrarian and funerary ceremonials.

As mentioned the appearance of the buttocks was symbolic of a death mask. The supple skin had been rendered lifeless, and the lower half of the torso was immobile, with the discolouration of a cadaver. The body had defeated her, but worse, it had defeated her mother.

The child ostensibly so willing and anxious to participate, believed she must continue to exercise, to please her mother. Since she could not resist the mother's domineering power driven animus, she did so. Although it seemed she still played the rôle of the obedient child, the inner rebellion had started, the body was changing to that of a woman. The breasts had developed, the buttocks were enlarging, the feminine spirit, together with an increase of feminine consciousness was emerging. She had already been aware of subversive thoughts of ease and repose, in the sun. There had undoubtedly been unconscious stirrings, the beckoning of procreative power, and with it the need to escape from the mother's vice-like grip. However ego consciousness did not have the strength of will power to resist. The rebellious shadow was waiting in the wings, biding its time to appear in the centre of the stage, and as it did so, the mask of death descended upon the buttocks. It is an outstandingly beautiful image of the Self's answer to the mother's monomania, and deep unconsciousness. The morphoea was a death mask against the mother's ambition.

After some two or three years of psychological support, the girl made an excellent response. She was not able to undertake competitive water sports again, but life flowered for her in a different and more meaningful way.

REFERENCES

1 Jung, C. G., Collected Works, Vol. II, para 348.
2 Onians, R. B., Origins of European Thought, p. 135, Cambridge University Press.
3 Ibid.
4 Ibid.

PART III

12

THE ARCHETYPAL BACKGROUND OF SKIN DISEASE

During the last two centuries, the various skin disorders have been subjected to group classification. Included are the varied eczemas, scaling disorders, bullous reactions, and lichenifications to name but a few. The commonest prevailing symptom is irritation, and the preponderant sign is invariably associated with inflammatory reaction. The latter is expected to appear to a greater or lesser extent in almost all cases. As has been observed the skin as one organ, covers the body like a closely fitting garment, and has the outer appearance of a singularly static nature. This is far removed from actuality.

The skin is in a constant state of flux, subject to continual transformation. The microscopic examination of normal histological skin structure leads to the salient observation that there is a matchless harmonious process of ordered cell division, maturation, growth and eventual death. This image is especially evident in the epidermis because of its unique nature. The beholder is at once seized by the inescapable thought that the soma is always disciplined towards the ultimate goal of an exquisitely finely tuned, and balanced order. The intrusion of a certain derangement occasioned by an inflammatory process or the chaos of malignancy is curiously alien because it is a total opposite to its innate nature. However the immediate invocation of reparatory powers tends to cast off, erupt out, seal off by occlusion, or transform the injurious, offensive imbalance.

The prime skin lesion of each disease process ultimately determines the differentiation into single individual entities, such as for example psoriasis or perhaps eczema. Enfolded in this classification is the conscious perception that the skin disease per se is an end in itself. However the inherent rhythmic transforming power, constantly manifesting eternal change in the skin, points to an equally valid alternative conclusion, that skin disease may be simply part of a process. The prime lesion, be it primordial vesicle, parakeratotic cell, or intradermal bulla, being the marker indicating an actual stage of a greater undefined ongoing transformative process. This would account for so many ambiguities in skin reaction, where it is difficult to be explicit as to exact diagnosis, and interpretation at a given time.

If the specific skin disorder, a symptom of the background change, is then considered to be a synchronistic event with psyche, as is so often perceived, it can only reflect the inner psychic energic state. The interruption of the cyclical rhythm of the skin itself, then mirrors the inner obstruction to the flow of psychic energy as a result of the presence of an unconscious psychic content. The psychic and physical energic changes may be regarded as two sides of the same phenomenon.

Irritation, as the result of the insidious presence of an irritant, of whatever nature, implies the presence of something which is "irritating". A psychic irritant also suggests "irritation", and indicates a state of emotionality. Inflammation as a process of change, includes ideas, sensations and perceptions of warmth, heat, and fire, and which are also co-existent with and indicative of emotional disturbance.

Throughout the presented case-material there is a constant immediacy of "fire". Even, as observed, where the skin has the semblance of death (as in lichen planus) "fire" is perceived in the early stages. Below the 'fieriness' is the brooding presence of unseen powers affecting the cyclical rhythm, transformation, rebirth and renewal of the organ. The two archetypes which are constantly present, and which preponderate in all cases of skin disease and disorder are those of fire and the serpent.

13

THE ARCHETYPE OF FIRE

Inflammation (Latin, inflammationem) means the action of inflaming or setting on fire, with the associative condition of being in flames. In somatic pathology it describes a morbid process characterized by heat, redness, swelling or pain.[1]

Inflammation occurs in all living tissues when attacked by antagonistic forces. It should result in regeneration because that is the goal towards which the body strives. Regeneration is the healing of damaged tissue so that it again presents the same form, which pre-existed the injury.

In dermatoses the classical signs of inflammation are visible. They are redness, resulting from increased blood flow from dilatation of the blood vessels. This produces a rise of temperature, and imparts a sensation of burning or heat. Swelling evolves from alteration of the fluid composition of the tissues. Pain accompanies the process and is described as burning, tingling, pricking or itching. Phrases deployed to describe these sensations include, 'hot', 'boiling', 'burning' or 'fiery'. All have associations to fire which appears to wind like a symbolic scintillating crimson ribbon of flame throughout most skin disease processes.

The degree of subjective sensation is variable being dependent on the actual disease process and the pain-threshold of the individual. To neutralize or abate the irritation of the pain, certain physical actions are recruited. The commonest is the reflex one of scratching, and to a slightly lesser extent the curious rhythmic reaction of rubbing. This is usually performed by the palmar pads of the fingers, and the soft tissues of the dominant hand, but any part of a member may be so employed.

The descriptive terms, used to describe both subjective and objective sensations, together with scratching, rubbing, friction, and blowing as physical acts of auto-pacification lead to the unavoidable conclusion that there is always the hidden presence of the archetype of fire in all morbid skin states.

Fire with its brightness, illumination and warmth is an integral part of all human life. In the West it was always regarded as an element, whereas in China fire was considered to be a phenomenon. It is both purifying and destructive and because of its inherent nature has occupied the minds of men for countless aeons.

The image of fire is found universally in myth. Hephaistos the Greek god was a smith, and the god of artistic creation. He was a master of the fire, and there are innumerable myths concerned with his being.

The image of fire and the fiery world has been well documented by Mircea Eliade in his book on Shamanism. Magic and magicians are to be found more or less everywhere, but only the shaman exhibits a particularly magical mastery over fire. The smiths of the Siberian, African and North American Indian tribes were the great medicine men, and spiritual rulers. This was so, because they could handle fire, and were entitled 'Master of Fire'. They performed all manner of fire acts or tricks[2] they could burn a man to ashes in the embers of the fire, and a few minutes afterwards the same man would be seen taking part in a dance, a great distance away.[3] Other fire acts included swallowing live coals, touching red hot iron or walking on fire. Mastery over fire implied that the master had acquired 'inner heat'. Mystical or inner heat was creative resulting "in a kind of magical power which creates".[4] Included for example are the creative acts of numerous illusions and miracles such as the negation of physical laws, and magical flight as performed by shamans and ascetics. "Fire" and "mystical heat" were connected with the ecstatic state indicating that the shaman had entered the realm of the Spirit world.

Von Franz in describing fire as libido or psychological energy especially in its emotional manifestations likens it to "Tapas", which is mentioned in the Rigveda. She explains that[5] "I have translated Tapas by 'brooding' because it is the only word in English which combines the two meanings of warmth and thought". Tapas is used in different Yoga schools, and means a specific form of meditation. Enfolded in all these ideas of fire, as connected with shamanism, and the medicine men, is the meaning of creation and production by means of fire.

The acquisition of fire by mankind was regarded as a theft, since it was the property of deity. Primitive peoples attributed the power of growth and of healing to an all pervading force which was generally called mana. It signified a hidden essence, a magical power, innate to all things. It corresponded to what, today is regarded as energy.

The ancient aborigines of Central Australia believed that the land of the Dreamtime or the Beyond consisted of "maiaurli" little soul sparks, which were the souls of the ancestors. This very ancient idea is found in many extremely primitive peoples. Jung[6] in enlarging upon the "maiaurli" explains that they were believed to be of a malicious nature, and inconvenient for women, if they happened not to be pregnant. It was the practice of these impish beings, to jump out of rocks, trees, lakes and rivers straight into the uterus of a woman, and if she had forgotten certain incantations, she at once conceived. In order to avoid such a mishap, a young woman pretended to be old and lame, so that the "maiaurli" were no longer interested. This ancient idea continued throughout the Middle Ages as the "scintilla", or soul spark.

Earlier Heraclitus,[7] the Ionic philosopher whose writings date five hundred years before Christ believed that the soul was "a spark of stellar essence". Saturninus[8] taught the same idea, which later came to be called the "scintilla vitae", the "little spark of the soul" or Seelenfünklein by Meister Eckhart.[9] Simon Magus[10] also believed that "semen and milk contained a very small spark", which increases and becomes a power, boundless and immutable.

It becomes clear that the ancient idea of the scintilla is related to the central point, the point which is the "centre of all things",[11] a God-image. It is an idea inherent in the symbolism of the mandala. Heraclitus called life itself "an ever-living fire". His ideas can be compared to the "primal warmth" of the Stoic philosophers and later with the phlogiston theory. This substance is defined as "a principle of inflammability formerly supposed to exist in combustible bodies".[12]

It was understood to be present in all things, as an invisible and hidden heat, also to be a principle of life. Jung[13] explains that phlogiston was "a certain quality of the unconscious which imparts the warmth of life". It is therefore, an inner phenomenon which may be experienced directly during an emotional condition such as the irruption of an irritable thought, as an outburst of anger, or as a blaze of furious rage. The ancients perceived it as the fiery substance of phlogiston incorporated in outer objects; it was not related by them to their own emotional being, it was a projection upon the external world.

In the writings of Jung, the archetype of fire is seen to play an outstanding rôle in alchemy. The epoch of alchemy persisted throughout seven centuries. It was practised mostly by physicians who worked in solitude. Jung's immense work over many years has brought to modern consciousness its forgotten existence, and by means of painstaking research into a multitude of alchemical treatises he was able to decipher and interpret the meaning inherent in alchemy. His remarkable discoveries enabled him to substantiate his concept of the collective unconscious. Therefore, no discussion of the archetype of fire would be complete without reference to Jung's findings, in this respect, and in particular the secret fire of the alchemists.

In modern civilised life a living fire is rarely seen nowadays, since wood and coal have been replaced by gas, oil and electricity, for heating and cooking. In the vast cities of the western world children no longer sit at their mother's knee, in front of a living fire. They miss the sound of the explosive crackling of combustible gases, the warmth and the sight of the leaping flames, their brightness, their colours and their beauty, with the accompanying showers of sparks. There is no longer the opportunity to fantasise, reflect, and meditate upon the creative flame, nor to realize its potential destructive nature. Fire no longer carries for them, the mystery and excitement inherent in the blaze. In this respect humanity has become the poorer, since severed from consciousness of the ongoing immediacy of the archetype.

The fire in alchemy was always kept alight, it was not permitted to go out, so that the goal of the opus could be achieved. This was to produce the elixir of life, an Alexipharmakon which neutralized poison, and cured mortal ills of the body. It increased the life span of man, and also promoted immortality. As a red tincture it cured sick nature, and as the lapis philosophorum, the philosophical stone, or stone of the wise, it cured illnesses of the soul, and mental diseases such as those which initiate melancholia and also madness.

Jung[14] says that "fire is in itself an uniter of opposites, and is a very ancient image of God". The same idea is implicit in the extracanoniacal saying of Christ[15] "Who is near to me is near to the fire. He who is far from me is far from the Kingdom". Jung explains[16] that the "inmost nature of Christ is fire, that everlasting fire which is the goal of alchemy". Later he[17] says, "the god Dionysos himself fits into this connection for his nature is also fire". Indeed as was the fiery breath of the pneuma.

There is a picture from the Rupertsberg Codex Scivias, written by Hildegard Von Bingen (12th Century)[18] depicting the quickening or the 'animation' of the Child in the body of His Mother. In the text Hildegard describes the souls of men as "fireballs". Jung[19] states that presumably the soul of Christ was also such a ball for Hildegard interprets her vision not with reference to the growth of a human child but with a particular reference to Christ, and the Mother of God.

In a text of the Musaeum Hermeticum[20] "The fire with which it is sublimated is called the fire of wisdom, and also a steaming fire". In explanation of this unusual description of fire, Jung[21] says that "a steaming fire is obviously not an ordinary fire" ... "but must be a mixture of fire and water, that is a mixture of the opposites" ... "wisdom is produced by a conflict of opposites". The alchemist, Khunrath[22] was to say of Sapientia "the salt of wisdom is a fire, yea a fire of salt".

In another very old treatise quoted by Jung it is mentioned where the house of wisdom is to be found. "The house stands in the belly of the earth, it can be perfected through the fire, and this is the perfecting of our wisdom."[23]

The fire with which wisdom is compared is the alchemical fire the ignis

179

noster, or the ignis occultus, the fire which was "our fire" or the "hidden fire". This is a symbolic fire, and as has been observed today would be described conceptually as psychic energy. Bearing in mind that fire is an ancient image of God, Christ described himself as fire, the Holy Ghost was seen to be fire, Sapientia is of the fire, and in its nefarious aspect it is Lucifer or Hell Fire. Von Franz[24] says "Flame or Fire as a widespread symbol for the soul, and as an image of psychic energy it seems to have been venerated in many primitive religions as something divine. It plays a central rôle in the religious life of those communities as the God image does in ours". She describes it as an archetypal idea of a cosmic divine energy capable of consciousness.

These ideas of the ancient alchemists may seem to be far removed from the modern concepts of medicine. Indeed they are, because, modern consciousness has lost contact with its roots in the unconscious world, and its archetypal structure. Therefore these ideas are strange, and appear irrational and irrelevant. They are nevertheless possessed of a living reality. The invisible fire so well known to the world of alchemy as their secret and hidden fire, remains as it always was, with its creative, and hellishly destructive aspects.

The soul of man is likewise unchanged, it is not sick, it is the modern conscious attitude of mind towards the unconscious instinctual realm that is out of order. The fiery world, and the fiery soul of man is derelicted, abandoned and lost to him.

In the appearance of a humble eczema of the face, an abject demeaning psoriasis of the knees, or a horrifying and mortal erythroderma, however the fire reappears, the soul reappears, and brings the transforming power with its divine potentiality, to enlarge consciousness in the individual sufferer, as part of the individuation process, or to lead downwards to hellish suffering through the subterranean fires into death.

The meaning of the fire therefore which includes all, from the highest passionate zeal of the Holy Ghost to the abominable hell and vile passions of Luciferian fire, is contained in the widely divergent extremes of affect and emotionality of which humanity is capable. These emotions are not normally visible in ordinary life, for they are unacceptable in social congress, therefore they are hidden or suppressed or are quite unconscious. Fire is thus the symbolical equivalent of an affect or a very strong and deep emotion. As has been observed in the material, the latter is either only partially conscious, or totally unconscious. It must therefore, in order to become visible, that is conscious, seek to present itself as a "fire" in the skin – the external organ. The skin as the primitive mind has always known acts thus as the reflector of the soul, it is its psychic mirror.

The horse like the fire is a symbol of energic forces. In discussing the horse as a fire symbol Jung says[25] that "there is a distinct fire symbolism in the mystic quadriga mentioned by Dio Chrysostom: the highest god always drives his chariot round in a circle. The chariot is drawn by four horses, and the outside horse moves very quickly. He has a shining coat (that is 'skin')[26] bearing on it the signs of the zodiac and its constellations." A note is very interesting, Jung[27] mentions a schizophrenic patient who declared that her horses had "half moons" under their skins "like little curls". The I Ching is supposed to have been brought to China by a horse that had the magic signs (the river map) on his coat (skin).[26] The skin of the Egyptian sky goddess, the heavenly cow, is dotted with stars, and the skin of the Mithraic Aion bears the signs of the zodiac. These examples indicate the skin's ability to convey or reflect the lights of the collective unconscious, the divine, or archetypal lights, the light of God, which signifies illumination and consciousness.

Legend always conceives the discovery of fire as a robbery. The great fire-bringers include Prometheus, Hephaistos, Christ, the Holy Ghost, Lucifer and Mercurius. All brought higher consciousness through feeling, warmth and insightful ideas. The Indian firebringer was Matarisvan, and the activity of fire making was referred to by the verb manthami,[28] which means to shake, to rub, to bring forth by rubbing. According to Kuhn,[29] the root was manth or math, which had the associated meanings to tear, or break off, to pluck and also to rob. The pramantha or fire stick used in manthana or fire sacrifice had a sexual aspect in India, the fire stick representing the male phallus, and the bored wood underneath the feminine yoni. Thus from the frictional action between the male and female, the fire was symbolically born from the genitals of the woman.

The pricking, boring, rubbing, and tearing actions upon the skin have in fact the same inner meaning. An example rests in a woman patient who was seized by a fearful compulsion. She suffered from a serious disorder of the central nervous system which deprived her of speech. She began to bore into her left nostril with her left forefinger a few weeks before her death. She would bore for several hours at a time, rubbing and shaking her finger as she did so. The whole upper face became red and inflamed, and was hot to the touch. She produced a deep ulcer, and eventually she bored into the underlying large vessels, and she haemorrhaged to death. It seemed that the boring was a frenetic effort to get at the truth, to seek and pick out a valuable morsel of knowledge. Undoubtedly it was also the way that fate decreed she should die.

Throughout the shamanistic world[30] spontaneous vocation and the desire for initiation usually involves a mysterious illness or perhaps a symbolic ritual of mystical death suggested by dismemberment of the body and renewal of the organs.

The Yamana neophytes[31] of Tierra del Fuego (Land of Fire) rub the skin of their faces until a new skin or even a third skin appears. This new skin is visible only to initiates. The idea behind this practice is for the old skin to disappear in order to make room for the new skin which is thin and translucent. In the first weeks the neophyte is observed by the experienced yékamush (medicine man) and when he 'sees' the new skin the initiant is accepted. He continues to rub harder and eventually his cheeks are covered with a fine and even more delicate skin. When extreme pain is felt to the touch, the initiatory process is complete. This is a form of flaying, and signifies a transformation from a worse state to a better. The initiant is as it were newly born into life of an higher order that is the higher stage of consciousness required of a medicine man.

Rubbing is a curious practice which involves the action of moving backwards and forwards over a surface with a certain amount of pressure and friction. Together with a host of other reactions, such as boring, scratching, nose picking, finger drumming, leg swinging or doodling, it symbolizes an obstruction to the flow of psychic libido occasioned by the presence of an unconscious content. It appears that the flow has been either obstructed, become sluggish or has deviated. Rubbing concentrates, on the area it "rubs up the fire", and increases the blood supply to the physical part. This unconscious reaction reflects the increase required in energic flow, to overcome the psychic blockage, and enlarge consciousness.

The archetype of fire with its image of age-old ideas and instinctual reactions appears in order to resolve the malady of the victim. It brings by way of the skin disease the heat, warmth, pain, and reactive reflex actions in an endeavour to guide the sufferer to a level of consciousness where the psychic difficulties are recognised. The fire as an enlightener signifies emotion. If there is no emotion there is neither life nor light for the victim. It is only through emotional interest or excitement that there is illumination and clarification of a psychic content. Emotion as we have observed is therefore the carrier of consciousness.

The entire disease process represents a symbolic fire making and the goal is consciousness and re-vivification, but alas, not usually achieved without suffering and its hidden partner, insight.

REFERENCES

1 Shorter Oxford English Dictionary, Oxford University Press, 1933.
2 Eliade, Mircea, Shamanism, p. 316 n. 74, Arkana.
3 Ibid.
4 Ibid., p. 412.
5 Von Franz, M-L, Creation Myths Lecture Course, p. 132.
6 Jung, C. G., Alchemy Lecture Course Vol. 2, p. 124, Printed by Karl Schippeer & Co. Zürich.
7 Jung, C. G., Collected Works, Vol. 14, para 42. n. 58, Routledge & Kegan Paul, London.

8 Jung, C. G., Collected Works Vol. 9, para 344, n. 141, Routledge & Kegan Paul, London.
9 Ibid., n. 140.
10 Ibid., n. 146.
11 Ibid., para 343.
12 Shorter Oxford English Dictionary.
13 Jung, C. G., Alchemy Lecture Course Vol. II, p. 124, Printed by Karl Schippeer & Co. Zürich.
14 Ibid., Vol. I, p. 82, Printed by Karl Schippeer & Co. Zürich.
15 Ibid. p. 94.
16 Ibid.
17 Jung, C. G., Alchemy Vol. I, p. 94 Printed by Karl Schippeer & Co. Zürich.
18 Jung, C. G., Collected Works, Vol. X, para 765, Routledge & Kegan Paul, London.
19 Ibid., para 766.
20 Jung, C. G., Alchemy Vol. II, p. 73 n. 12. Museum Hermeticum Treatise lll p. 90. Printed by Karl Schippeer & Co. Zürich.
21 Ibid., p. 73.
22 Ibid., p. 76 n. 21 Khunrath M Von Hylealischen Chaos p. 229.
23 Ibid., p. 77 n. 23 Allegories Sapientum Supra Librum Turbae Theatrium Chemicum V l622 p. 67.
24 Von Franz, M-L, Aurora Consurgens p. 166 Routledge & Kegan Paul, London.
25 Jung, C. G., Collected Works, Vol. V, para 423, Routledge & Kegan Paul, London.
26 Author's comment.
27 Jung, C. G., Collected Works Vol. V, para 423, n. 21, Routledge & Kegan Paul, London.
28 Ibid., para 208.
29 Ibid. n. 5.
30 Eliade, Mircea Shamanism, Chap. 2, p. 53, Arkana.
31 Ibid., p. 53 n. 58.

14

THE ARCHETYPE OF THE
SERPENT

The organ of the skin by means of its inherent transformative powers, its ability to cast and regenerate itself unceasingly, is the symbolic 'snake' of the human body. In patients suffering from skin maladies the serpent often appears in dreams fantasies and even in reality as was seen in the case of the serpent girl with urticaria.

A middle aged man had what was thought to be a trifling ailment, accompanied by a feeling of malaise, and melancholic sadness. His physical condition appeared to be without cause for alarm, but because of the depression he came for psychological advice. Upon enquiry he produced an initial dream, which was however of a disturbing nature. He recited the dream in a matter of fact way with little evidence of any emotional reaction. In the dream he had perceived an image of a large black cobra before his eyes, with its hood raised, moving towards him in a threatening fashion. That was the dream.

When asked what he thought or felt about this image, he said it appeared as if the snake was going to attack him. He did not feel afraid but he did not care for the look of the snake. It was this lack of spontaneous reaction to the dark image which was so disturbing. Within a few weeks he became seriously ill, and sadly he died within a matter of months.

The dream portrayed the archetypal image of the serpent in its negative and potentially destructive aspect. The serpent as an animate autonomous being had undoubtedly intruded into his life and posed a grave threat. If he had encountered a cobra in reality he would have been both fascinated by its presence, and terrified of its potency. He would most probably have sought the means either to escape or protect himself. Because it was a dream cobra he was unable to equate its equivalent reality to that of an outer snake, and consequently felt no fear. But the inner cobra, albeit a dream image, was psychically real, it was a psychic fact, and the consequences of its ignored potential danger were the same for him. He was possessed of a fine intellect, with a rational cast of mind. Herein lay the danger, because his intuitive-feeling side was undeveloped he was unable to accept the reality of objective psyche. This lack of relationship towards the inner world of his own being had not permitted him to be equipped to experience the true meaning of the serpentine image which had appeared in the night to threaten him, and indeed, his life.

The serpent is a cold blooded chthonic animal which lives in crevices in the ground, or in holes below the earth. It is normally shy and timid, constantly avoiding man and only becoming dangerous if its person or its habitat is threatened. I once asked a Mayan Indian in Yucatan if it was true that rattlesnakes do not attack the North American Indian. He answered that he did not know, but thought that it was probably true. He said quite simply "They, (the Indians) like us, know where to put their feet and do not tread carelessly upon their brother's home". The appearance of the snake is always unexpected, it comes as a sudden intrusion (as it did in the dream), bringing with it heart-stopping fear for the observer.

The head of the snake is the focus, upon which attention is always riveted, with the brilliant eye and the constant flickering tongue. The sinuous movement of the muscular body encompasses both the upward spiral movement of vegetal growth and the propulsive and retrogressive motility of the animal body. The combination of the stillness of the head, the fixity of the stare, and the slow undulant writhing of the body is both hypnotic and terrifying. The fear engendered by its unexpected presence is of all that is unrelated and non-human. It reflects that which is dark, unclear, and obscure, belonging to the profound depths of the submarine and subterranean realms. The snake as we shall see, includes everything outside the range of human conscious awareness, from the Gnostic Agathodaimon at the highest level to the inferior devils of the lower orders.

The dream image of the cobra with its upraised hood is reminiscent of the figurative representations from ancient Egypt where the serpent was the most revered of animals. The hooded cobra was part of the head-dress of the Pharoahs signifying sovereignty of deity. The Egyptian Apophis serpent symbolized both light and darkness, as well as evil. The serpent's dark nature represented the principle of femininity. All the ancient goddesses of the Mediterranean basin either carried serpents, or snakes were wound round their arms heads or bodies. The plumed serpent of Pre-Columbian America (Quetzalcoatl) represented the synthesis of two opposing principles, as the great god he brought prosperity and culture to the Mesa-American civilization. In dry and arid Mexico, Tlaloc the rain god was a serpent. Coatlicue the great mother or earth goddess of Mexico was composed of serpents. She symbolized the earth, herself, and represented her devouring and deadly aspect. One of the effigies of the goddess discovered under the parvis of the cathedral in Mexico City about a century ago, depicts exactly the essential nature of this goddess. Her head is composed of the heads of two intertwined rattlesnakes, and her body is girdled by snakes, and skulls. One senses something hidden, cold, and extremely unnerving in this hideous image. It is the dark mother of Mexico's earth, that land of aridity, drought and volcanic fire. She carries a crushing and devouring power, whilst demanding obligatory sacrifice. This is the earth as the devouring mother, to whom all life returns, but also, from whom it is derived. As serpent she represents the spirit of ambiguity of the chthonic world which is that of transformation, enfolding birth, death, and renewal.

In retrospect the psychological meaning of the patient's dream image becomes apparent. The intrusion into the patient's life of the black cobra represents a dark chthonic principle of pure unconscious nature. To the conscious mind it is both antagonistic and dangerous. The presence of the upraised hood indicates the intention to kill. The serpent brings with its alien atmosphere, the breath of the underworld. It is as such an emissary of death for the physical body, against which ego is powerless.

The snake because of its ability to cast its skin came to symbolize the rejuvenation of nature in springtime, and thus it signified the eternal return, and immortality. Its chthonic nature, as has been seen, is associated with the souls of the departed. The idea being that the dead lived on in the underground after burial, in the form of snakes. It seemed that the dead man turned into a living snake, and the latter turned into the soul of the dead man. The souls of the Greek heroes were snakes, Erechtheus and Cecrops the founder of the Acropolis were worshipped in the forms of snakes. Heroes had snake eyes since they had snake souls. Of the exchange between man and snake Jung[1] says that "it is as if the potentiality for such an exchange were an attribute of the God, his revealed aspect being loving and spiritual, but then changing to another aspect which is both monstrous and horrible". To the primitive mind the snake represented the carrier of the mana of the spirit of the dead as well as the ever renewing vitality of life. Because of these associative ideas snake oracles and cults flourished world-wide.

Asklepios the god of healing and of physicians is believed to have arisen out of the earlier centuries of the millennium which preceded the Christian era, but may be far older, since temples were established at least three thousand years ago. The tenacious adoration of this well loved, widely revered and worshipped god was relinquished only with difficulty in favour of Christ and the new Christian religion.

The legend went through a strange metamorphosis in Greek mythology. First he seems to have been a mortal physician later an oracular daemon, and lastly an Apollonion deity. He was a god-hero, a mediator, a saviour and a messiah figure. Like all heroes, he had the soul of a serpent. He was regarded as a serpent god for he was in fact a serpent, being called the serpent, or the old serpent. At first his human representations revealed a dark demonic figure, which was superceded in later centuries first as a young virile man, and latterly as a benevolent fatherly figure. As the serpent he was also often portrayed in the form of the creature. The snake, which was invariably wound round his arm his person or a staff, which he carried, was also the god. The essential aspect of his worship was the incubatio. The worshipper underwent a therapeutic introversion, in the asklepeian or sanctuary of the temple. During this period he waited for a dream to bring about the transformation. The dream image of the god in human or serpentine form was the harbinger of healing.

The advent of the real snake into the life of the school teacher with urticaria after a period of deep introversion is a modern illustration of this age-old belief and therapy, which re-appears in the living archetype. The cure for the girl was a realization of herself as a woman willing to take responsibility for her own life. The serpent signified the release of a quantum of psychic energy from the grip of the maternal archetype. It was this newly acquired libido which was available to initiate the subsequent enlargement of consciousness and transformation of personality.

As the Christian religion overcame its rivals and increased in power, Christ himself was interpreted as a serpent because "he came mysteriously out of the darkness".[2] The Gnostics also favoured the serpent because it was a long standing and well established symbol for "the 'good' genius loci the Agathodaimon"[3] as was also the case with the Asklepian serpent. Christ shares the symbol of the serpent with the devil. As Jung reminds us, "Lucifer, the Morning Star means Christ as well as the devil."[4]

When a theriomorphic symbol makes its appearance in a dream or as an unconscious manifestation it depicts the psychic level of the unknown, unconscious content. It is as if the content is at a stage of unconsciousness that is as far away from the consciousness of a human being as would be the psyche of an animal. One can relate to a warm-blooded cat, and possibly in certain circumstances to a tiger, but it is impossible ever to relate to a snake. "The snake does in fact symbolize "cold blooded" inhuman contents and tendencies of an abstractly intellectual as well as concretely animal nature, in a word the extrahuman quality in man".[5]

In discussing the point of greatest tension between the opposites such as masculine and feminine, good and evil conscious and unconscious, Jung[6] emphasises the double significance of the serpent which is at the centre. "Being an allegory of Christ as well as the devil it contains and symbolizes the strongest polarity into which the Anthropos falls when he descends into Physis". He concludes[7] that "the ordinary man has not yet reached this point of tension: he has it merely in the unconscious, i.e in the serpent". In a footnote:[8]

187

"Most people do not have sufficient range of consciousness to become aware of the opposites inherent in human nature. The tensions they generate remain for the most part unconscious, but can appear in dreams. Traditionally the snake stands for the vulnerable spot in man; it personifies his shadow, i.e his weakness and unconsciousness. The greatest danger about unconsciousness is proneness to suggestion. The effect of suggestion is due to the release of an unconscious dynamic, and the more unconscious this is, the more effective it will be. Hence the ever-widening split between conscious and unconscious, increases the danger of psychic infection and mass psychosis. With the loss of symbolic ideas the bridge to the unconscious has broken down. Instinct no longer affords protection against unsound ideas and empty slogans. Rationality without tradition and without a basis in instinct is proof against no absurdity."

In the case history of the woman who lost her hair after the murderous attack by her husband, she had a fantasy that a black snake was curled up in her back. She knew that this was not a real snake, but she felt it was there. She always maintained that when the snake moved upwards the hair would grow. In fact it did do so eventually. The woman had a serious shadow problem, and since she had no conception of it, in consciousness, it was in fact the snake behind her back. Her range of consciousness was too inadequate for her to perceive her own opposite. The inner problem which was presented to her by way of a recurrent dream over a period of seven months appeared to point the finger at the outer mother-in-law, the mother of the murderous husband, who was in fact a witch. Undoubtedly this was an outer reality, but the equivalent shadow problem of the woman herself was that which was vital for her own individuation process. It was at this point, when the unconscious posed the problem to her that she said that the black snake in her back had moved to a higher level. This intimated that the unconscious psychic content had moved to a stratum where there was a possibility of experiencing it emotionally, and the possibility, although remote, of assimilation into consciousness.

The woman had lived a protected life since her marriage, she had allowed herself to be fully dependent on her husband's largesse. Then he turned against her and in the night he tried to kill her with their children. The fearful shock and the ensuing panic-fear of finding herself alone without a future, although it indubitably came from the actual situation, also issued from the craven fear of the instinctual unconscious inner shadow woman, who was, at a blow, deprived of everything that she held dear. She had forgotten her dependence on the unconscious in the years of her security. She had turned her back on its instinctual wisdom, and the fantasy in the form of a black snake in her back gripped her. This snake was a symbol of the unconscious possession, her bewitchment. In the end she was unable to perceive her inner avenging nature, and therefore could not relinquish it. Her own unconscious then rode, like a demon-serpent, on her back acting as a brake to her conscious development.

The fantasy of the black snake which beset her, entered her life as suddenly as a real snake would come into her garden. For centuries the snake has been used as a symbol of the unconscious. The snake itself is really a spinal column and was used by the Gnostics as a symbol for the spinal cord and the basal ganglia. Jung said that "if the unconscious be localised anywhere it is in the basal ganglia . . . the snake really represents the vegetative psyche, the basis of the instincts".[9]

The upward movement, or the ascent of the black snake in the woman's fantasy recalls to mind the activation of the Kundalini serpent or the serpent fire of Indian Tantric philosophy. The object of which is to enable the arousal of the goddess by a method of intense introverted concentration on the part of the Tantric yogins. The energic serpent power will be released and through penetration of the successive chakras or centres will eventually mount to unite with the god Shiva, the Lord of Light or Consciousness. Shakti as the goddess of primordial energy is symbolized as a snake coiled at the bottom of the spinal cord in the pelvic area, three and a half times round the lingam. Each chakra in the ascent is the representation of a stage in the evolution of consciousness. The lowest region is the muladhara, the perineum, at the base of a small basin. The next is the water region of the bladder at the entrance of the basin. The third region is the abdominal centre, and is called the fire region corresponding to the solar plexus, were one can perceive certain emotions. This is as far as the snake ascended in the woman's fantasy. It did not reach the next stage, the feeling centre so she was not able to reflect upon her psychic situation. The fantasy snake settled down at a level below the diaphragm and did not ascend any higher at that time. The woman remained possessed by her vengeful shadow, of which she was totally unconscious.

The shadow is probably the most powerful of all archetypes, and is potentially the most dangerous, because it has very deep connections with evolutionary history, and contains much of mans' basic animal nature. By 'shadow', one means the inferior personality, the lowest levels of which correspond to the instinctual nature of the animal world. Jung[10] says "since the shadow itself is unconscious for most people the snake would correspond to what is totally unconscious and incapable of becoming conscious, but which, as the collective unconscious and as instinct, seems to possess a peculiar wisdom of its own, and knowledge that is often felt to be supernatural".

In alchemy the serpent played an immense rôle symbolically. The Ouroboros was seen as a snake devouring its tail, it became the symbol of the alchemical work of transformation as a circular self contained process. The alchemists conceived Mercurius, as the spirit of alchemy and the Mercurial serpent or serpens mercurialis, the chthonic spirit who dwelt in mat-

189

ter especially the original chaos hidden in creation, the massa confusa. Mercurius was closely identified with the immensely archaic Greek god of mediators. Hermes with his serpent entwined caduceus was the eternal, bewitching, beguiling constant deceiver, yet, always a bringer of good things to men. This god of prophecy, and revelation as the mercurial serpent in the fire, is the light bringer, but is not himself the light.

As has been seen the snake symbol in alchemy developed from earlier images, one is not unmindful of the snake in the Garden of Eden. The conception of Mercurius was that in the form of a snake he lived in the earth, he had a body, soul and spirit. Jung[11] says "He was believed to have a human shape, as the homunculus or homo altus and was regarded as the earthly God". Later Jung[12] has this to say "As serpens mecurialis the snake is not only related to the god of revelation Hermes, but as a vegetative numen calls forth the 'blessed greenness' all the budding and blossoming of plant life. Indeed this serpent dwells even in the interior of the earth and is the pneuma that lies hidden in the stone". The stone as the stone of the wise, the lapis philosophorum is the goal of the alchemical process. Mercurius as the serpent is a healer, he is a mediator that is a peacemaker, like Hermes.

He is also "a servator" or "preserver of the world" and a "salvator" a "healer of imperfect bodies".[13] Mercurius has the circular nature of the ouroboros and is symbolized by a circle of which he is also the centre. He is able to say of himself "I am One and at the same time Many in myself".[14]

Here is an example of the insidious intrusion of the serpens mercurialis into the life of a modern individual.

Some years ago a middle aged man was referred for dermatological advice. At the time he was undergoing chaemotherapy for a severe depressive psychosis, and had been hospitalized for over half a year. The condition obligating referral was an excoriated self-inflicted skin disease of the legs. His psychiatric advisors were at a loss as how to treat his condition since the self mutilation was both severe and uncontrollable.

The man was of average height, nondescript in appearance, severely underweight, and looked much older than his years. His eyes, clouded behind uncleaned spectacle frames, were blue in colour, lifeless and unfocussed. He was dressed in the standard pyjamas and dressing gown supplied by the hospital authorities. We exchanged the usual courtesies, and without demur he sat down and began to tear at the skin of the legs. There was neither preamble nor explanation. It appears, and this later proved to be so, that his visit to me was an interference in the act of tearing the skin.

The action of the hands was singularly hypnotic in that the finger nails, though short were plunged deep into the flesh, and then as he flexed his arms, they moved upwards, leaving four parallel gouges on each leg from the upper part of the foot to the infrapatellar areas of the knees. The action was rhythmic and took place several times each minute. After several deep scratches he changed his position slightly without altering the steady rhythm

190

of the claw-like hands. The skin covering the legs had been completely stripped off leaving each leg, denuded, exposing a gory mass of underlying flesh. The facial expression showed neither pain nor discomfort. His hands were covered in blood and his finger nails encrusted with inspissated serum and blood. Whilst he mutilated himself no word was spoken. In the silence the only sound to be heard was the scraping of the nails on the skin, and an occasional plop, as a drop of blood dripped on to the floor.

My initial reaction was one of horrified dismay as I sat silently with him and observed the macabre nature of his actions. There was nothing to be said in such a circumstance, and I had no idea what to do. An inspiration came to me, and I arranged for some childrens' modelling plasticine to be brought in for him. Within a quarter of an hour it was available. I gave the material to him, and suggested that instead of wounding himself he was to make things with his hands. I spoke to him as if it was the most natural thing for a human being to sit silently, and literally tear himself to pieces. His legs were dressed, and he departed.

Three days later he returned with the blood stained bandages hanging off, but he was not tearing himself with quite the same intensity as before. He had done nothing with the modelling clay. The instructions were re-issued in the same matter-of-fact way, and again bandages were applied to the legs as protection.

Three days later he returned, but this time the dressings were in-situ and he had a different facial expression. He seemed more alert. Underneath his arm he carried a cardboard box from which he extracted a few clay models. The material originally had consisted of several colours. The man had rolled them altogether, and the resulting amalgam was a muddy brown colour. He had modelled some blob-like shapes which had the appearance of squatting, each had eyes and a mouth. Undoubtedly they were quite hideous, and so I enquired what they were. At the precise moment I asked the question there was a tremendous crash behind me, and one of the assistant nurses who was pregnant, fainted and fell full length on the floor. I got up to investigate, and so did the patient. He suddenly spoke, remarking "What is the matter with her?" and I told him that his models had frightened her, whereupon a pleased look flitted across his face, and he agreed it was probably so, because they also frightened him.

He then went on to explain that the models were in fact 'gremlins'. He had served in the Royal Air Force during the Second World War, and the air crews ad ground staff used to speak of gremlins constantly. They are little mischievous imps, quite invisible, which get into the aeroplane engines, or the aeroplanes themselves plaguing and tricking the airmen.

That day marked the first turning point for afterwards he began to speak to me, not exactly freely but he would often utter, several sentences at a time. However from that day it was clear that he had begun to take a great interest in his creations. As he arrived in the clinic he always explained the finer points of his work. At first the models consisted of formless shapes, but slowly they began to change and took upon themselves various serpentine forms. The colours of the plasticine remained disagreeable and unchanged because he used it over and over again.

He was seen weekly and as soon as the serpentine forms appeared, he stopped mutilating himself. Because his hands had been freed from their compulsive actions he began to produce quantities of models, which he started to bring in a plastic carrier bag. The snakes were of every shape, and size, in all kinds of attitudes, some were coiled up, others elongated, whilst some were zig-zag in shape, and so on. He always placed them with great care on the surface of my desk. I realized quite early on that I was really witnessing the Ouroboros as a circular self-contained process, and the plasticine was indeed the prima material. It became clear also in time that he produced on the desk surface a concrete image of the psychic dissociation with the scattered undirected, apparently purposeless psychic libido.

It was very strange to watch the same pattern week after week. He always placed the snakes on the desk with the same exactly precise gestures as if he was placing a priceless jewel, which in fact he was so doing.

As time passed I began to be aware that the snakes had taken upon themselves definite forms, as pythons, mambas, cobras, and boa constrictors took over the desk surface.

After two months it was evident that the legs had healed and since his depression had also improved, together with his psychic awareness, his psychiatric advisors decided to discharge him. Although he was most certainly no longer a dermatological invalid, I decided not to discharge him, and suggested that he continue with his work visiting me once a month to show me what he had done. He agreed and some weeks later about three or four months after the initial visit, he arrived with his bag.

Again he produced a collection of muddy-brown snakes, but surprisingly each was fitted with a diamond collar. He explained that he had visited a department store and had bought a cheap diamond necklace such as young girls buy. (It was in fact a paste pseudo-diamanté necklace). From it, he made a little collar for each of his snakes. This act apparently both 'collared' the energy, and also gave to it the highest value. It also revealed his intense conscious interest and the energy now available to ego, in the procuration and fashioning of the collars.

The word diamond is derived from the Greek word, adamant, which means invincible and unconquerable. A diamond like all precious stones symbolizes treasure, it is the hardest of stones (immortal) signifying light (conscious illumination) life and purity. Mircea Eliade[15] has related diamonds to 'snake stones' which in many colours, are thought to have fallen from the heads of snakes and dragons. There is also a widespread folk belief that they are derived from the spittle of snakes. In the Middle East there is a belief that diamonds are poisonous, if permitted to touch the lips, because they once had been in snakes' throats. The diamond is also linked with the supreme female deity which is usually associated with the earth. In Tibet the earth goddess Tara has a human incarnation, the "Diamond Sow".

The patient declared when he brought the collared snakes, "I thought those snakes would look nice in diamond collars". By this simple phrase he exposed an air of proprietorship and at the same time there was a suggestion that they were of the feminine gender, although there was nothing concrete to substantiate this impression. He himself made no other comment.

A few months later he came again this time with a charming smile, and on arrival he said immediately "You will be pleased with this!" When he produced it from the bag, there was only a single snake. It was about five or six inches in length rearing up like a cobra, and on its head was a golden crown – it was a crowned serpent. I told him I was pleased indeed, because it was so beautiful, and it was, both beautiful and extraordinary. (He had made the crown from a little golden ring.)

This wonderful transformation occurred about six months after the onset of the dermatological disorder. He was by that time completely discharged from psychiatric care and was living at home with his wife. He was well, and as he had retired from work prior to the psychiatric illness, therefore he decided to house-keep for his wife as she had become unwell. He was able to live on a state pension supplemented by his retirement pension from work.

He and I decided that we should continue to observe his work and he would visit me every three months to show me the products of his creativity. I myself wished to follow this strange pattern of healing, which was entirely spontaneous.

After the appearance of the crowned serpent, the man gave up modelling clay. He began to read books which he had never had time to do before, and to take walks in the country. Then again quite suddenly and spontaneously he began to draw, using a pencil at first and then a pen. He only very rarely and much later used colour. Eventually he brought the drawings for me to see, and I was astonished at their arresting nature. A bundle was produced every three or six months over a period of five years. During that time he produced several hundreds of pictures, all of an extremely high standard revealing an artistic talent of considerable quality, with very fine draughtsmanship. He had never done anything like it before in his life.

Strangely, however, every single drawing was of a young woman. All the girls which he drew were dressed in clothes of the period of the nineteen twenties – known as "the twenties", the decade which followed on immediately after the Great War of 1914–1918. That was the period in England when women obtained the right to vote, and it was a turning point in feminine emancipation.

The young women of the drawings were quite simply, sensational. They

193

were all of a certain type, young with fashionably bobbed hair of the day. Often the hair was kept in place by a diamanté or bejewelled bandeau round the forehead. The dresses were short, of the tunic type and many of the girls wore the modish cloche or bell hats, with long scarves or feather boas. Frequently they were either smoking (which was very avant garde in those days) or a glass of wine was held in the hand. Sometimes they were either getting into, or out of racing cars, with pieces of luggage usually strewn about. That was the theme, it depicted in great detail the essential, young, modern, liberated seductress of the time. As I gazed at the multitude of girls, it was like watching a film of those days. Here was a woman 'ready to travel'.

The patient was sixty years old, almost as old as the century so the twenties represented the time of his youth. It was truly astounding to see how he had captured those gestures, and attitudes of that fashionable world, the world of the glittering, giddy, madcap years of champagne, fizz, flappers (the name given to the girls) and all the 'bright young things'. Of course it was a world he had never known, but he had caught and drawn its essence exactly. The girls in spite of their beauty, all were beautiful and carefree, were also haughty with a distinct imperiousness of attitude. This was the opposite demeanour to that of the patient. He was colourless, taciturn, rather seedy in appearance. His clothes though neat and clean never seemed to fit him. This gave him a slightly grotesque, and distinctly Chaplinesque air which was always present. It was difficult, to believe that he was the artist of these lovely girls, but he was, and they were images of an aspect of his 'lady soul'.

When the explosion of energy had died away he did no more in the way of creative work. He was obliged to care for his wife, until she died eventually. This he did admirably, and he also weathered a multitude of difficulties in his private life. He had to learn to live alone and care for himself. In later years he was accompanied by a lively young grand-daughter, previously he had always come alone. Apart from his war service he had never lived outside the town where he was born. He had worked as a clerk, for the civil service all his life, until he was forced against his will to retire at 60 years of age, it was after this that the psychosis intervened. In all he attended my practice for fifteen years and came always punctually and regularly. He never had another psychotic episode and he lived his life bravely after his recovery. There was never any question of analysis which would have been quite impracticable.

This was a most unusual and informative case. It was a modern day alchemical opus, in which a transformation of psychic energy occurred bringing with it, sanity, and an increased consciousness, with a stability of personality, forged throughout an intense and prolonged period of introversion and creativity. The process to watch was outstanding, both he and I were gripped with the events. Here was the fire, the emotionality on his part, and the excitement, curiosity and amazement on mine. The culmina-

194

tion was the advent of the crowned serpent at the end of the serpentine phase. Then came the 'éclatement' of the anima, all that unlived life. She had undoubtedly been sleeping for all of his life, and suddenly she awoke, and the excitement was tangible.

The act of tearing away at the skin and the flesh of the legs was in fact a flaying, with a suggestion of dismemberment. This, as has been seen, is a transformation symbol signifying renewal and rebirth. The legs as pillars of the body represented the whole support of his masculine corporeal being, and were it seemed in urgent need of renewal. The hands produced the snake pit, which underwent a transformation when the formless libido was contained in the serpentine shape, and eventually 'collared', that is domesticated. It was then no longer dangerous, the psychic dissociation was in the act of being controlled. The advent of the crowned serpent brought healing and complete resolution of the illness.

In the serpent itself one associates the Asklepian, the Mercurial, and the Agathodaimon serpents of antiquity, and alchemy. The golden crown on the serpent's head indicated that it was of the highest value. The numinous and disturbing appearance of the unusual image was at once reminiscent of the Agathodaimon serpent of Greek antiquity portrayed on Gnostic gems with a seven or twelve rayed crown.

Agathodaimon was an important Greek god as the good spirit of the cornfields and the vineyards he was also the protector of both the individual and the State. He was portrayed usually in the form of a snake, sometimes as a young man, a shepherd, holding a poppy pointing downwards in one hand, and a wheat ear in the other pointing upwards. This revealed the two aspects of the symbol, although he was reputed to be the bringer of good fortune and good health, and life. He was oracular as well as a teacher of wisdom. His full name resolves into the "resplendent sole one" – the sun. The snake represents the cold ruthless instinctuality of the dark world of the instincts, but as noted contains natural wisdom also, hence goodness, light and healing are embodied in the archetype. The Agathodaimon plays an especially important rôle in alchemy, where he is represented as a serpent. Jung[16] draws attention to a remarkable quotation from Ostanes in Abu'l'Qasim describing the intermediate position between two pairs of opposites constituting a quaternio.

"Ostanes said, Save me, O, my God for I stand between two exalted brilliances known for their wickedness and between two dim lights; each of them has reached me and I know not how to save myself from them. And it was said to me, Go up to Agathodaimon the Great and ask aid of him, and know that there is in thee somewhat of his nature which will never be corrupted. . . . And when I ascended into the air he said to me, Take the child of the bird which is mixed with redness and spread for the gold of its bed which comes forth from the glass, and place it in its vessel whence it has no power to come out except when thou desirest and leave it until its moistness has departed".

Ostanes it seems is a diversity of persons instead of one, he is dissociated. "It is presumably Hermes who points out to Ostanes that something incorruptible is in his nature which he shares with Agathodaimon, something divine, obviously the germ of unity."[17]

It seems that this central germ is the alchemical gold, the aurum philosophorum, or the gold of the opus and the philosophers. It is also the hermetic bird which must be entrapped in the hermetic vase, sealed and heated until all moisture that is unconsciousness is evaporated. Therefore as Jung points out, some kind of consciousness is apparently indicated. Another part of the same text is interesting, where Hermes says to the Sun: "I cause to come out to thee the spirits of thy brethren (the planets) O, Sun and I make them for thee a crown the like of which was never seen; and I cause thee and them to be within thee and I will make thy Kingdom vigorous".[18] The crown signifies kingly totality and it represents unity, which is resistant to splitting apart. Jung points out that the Agathodaimon serpent wears such a crown in Gnostic gems, as does Wisdom in the Aurora Consurgens.

The appearance of the golden crowned serpent in the patient's exposition of the material confirmed the goal of the long and arduous journey in the dangerous underworld. He had arrived at the central place, the house of the inner ruler, the Lord (the Self) of that realm who had initiated the process, transformed it and completed it, and who was also the process itself.

The subsequent five years during which he drew endlessly, images of the anima, was a period of unexampled vigour and energy. It was the energic force of the unlived feminine which had lain dormant for forty years, until released. There is little doubt that in spite of all his external difficulties, he did enjoy himself in this creative period, when he found great fulfilment. After the advent of the sparkling and fiery anima it became quite evident that he had at last begun to relate to other patients, assistants, and the accompanying small grand-daughter.

The whole episode is a beautiful example of a transformation from madness to sanity, in which one perceived the awakening of the soul, and the entrance of Eros into the life of a middle aged man. The gateway was the lowly skin disease which appeared to ignite the conflagration, but was after all the mirrored image of the psychic fire, and chaotic destruction.

A word about the unconscious may be fitting at this point as a reminder. Jung[19] said these fine words

"The collective unconscious is anything but an encapsulated personal system; it is sheer objectivity, as wide as the world and open to all the world. There I am the object of every subject, in complete

196

reversal of my ordinary consciousness, where I am always the subject that has an object. There I am utterly one with the world, so much a part of it, that I forget all too easily who I really am 'Lost in oneself' is a good way of describing this state. But this self is the world, if only a consciousness could see it. That is why we must know who we are".

From these examples there is ample confirmation of the outstanding rôle of the serpent archetype in dermatological disorder.

REFERENCES

1 Jung, C. G., The Visions Seminars, Vol. 2, p. 345, Spring Publications, Switzerland.
2 Jung, C. G., Collected Works, Vol. 9, 11 para 291, Routledge & Kegan Paul, London.
3 Ibid.
4 Ibid., para 127.
5 Jung, C. G., Collected Works, Vol. 9, 11 para 291, Routledge & Kegan Paul, London.
6 Ibid., para 390.
7 Ibid.
8 Ibid. n. 79.
9 Jung, C. G, Alchemy, Vol. I, p. 116, Printed by Karl Schippeer & Co. Zürich.
10 Jung, C. G., Collected Works, Vol. 9, 11 para 370, Routledge & Kegan Paul, London.
11 Ibid., para 367.
12 Ibid., para 386.
13 Jung, C. G., Collected Works, Vol. 13, para 283, Routledge & Kegan Paul, London.
14 Ibid., para 280.
15 Eliade, Mircea, Patterns in Comparative Religions, New York 1958.
16 Jung, C. G., Collected Works, Vol. 14, Mysterium Coniunctionis, para 5, Routledge & Kegan Paul, London.
17 Ibid., para 6.
18 Ibid.
19 Jung, C. G., Collected Works, Vol. 9, 1 para 46, Routledge & Kegan Paul, London.

PART IV

EPILOGUE

EPILOGUE

The primitive mind has always equated the skin with the soul. The modern mind, conditioned by rational intellectualism and seduced by the brilliant wizardry of modern technology no longer considers the soul of man to be of relevance. It is caught in the firm belief that there is a rational explanation for everything and that all physical disease must have a somatic cause. Furthermore it also believes that it is simply the continuation of ever-deeper probing researches into the physical structure and metabolism of the body, which will eventually uncover the underlying causation of all things.

It is quite understandable that the modern intellect by virtue of its single-mindedness finds it difficult to accept an aetiological viewpoint other than causal, because it is based strictly on lineal thinking. However since psyche is not just composed of a rational consciousness, but also an irrational unconscious there is therefore a place for an altogether different approach to the problem.

It has been the endeavour of this work to portray as clearly as is possible the central rôle of unconscious psyche in the aetiology of skin disease. Undeniably, physical changes are almost always present but they appear to be 'symptoms' as it were, of the unknown and therefore unrecognised psychic disorder. It is important to remember that unconscious psyche is unconscious.

The nature of the skin itself must be considered. It is an organ consisting of five layers which constantly sheds and renews itself throughout life. It is therefore an organ of transformation, which is always changing, yet ever remaining the same. It is also a model of exquisite harmony in the healthy state. For the subject the skin is the organ of demarcation from the external world, beyond is 'other' and alien, ego-conscious awareness of selfhood ends at the skin. As a reflector of the inner somatic state its variations are dependent upon the ebb and flow of the vascular supply. If diminished or depleted in some measure automatic changes in colour and humidity occur. Thus any change in the health or the emotional life of the subject, is immediately visible.

When a disease invades the normal process of skin change, the natural goal, which is balanced equilibrium, is disrupted. The histological appearance suggests that in spite of the blockage occasioned by the primary lesion, of whatever nature, the continual transforming process aims to cast off, seal, or occlude the "intrusive agent". This leads to the concept that the skin disease is symptomatic of a disruption of the energic flow. It seems that the skin reflects, not a physical but a psychic disorder.

The abandoned or neglected psyche in order to demonstrate its presence and draw attention to its plight must attract the attention of ego-consciousness through the mediation of the skin. The frequently observed archetypal images of the preponderant archetypes, substantiate this theorem. That of fire is indicative of emotionality as a potential increase of consciousness, and the serpent is symbolic of objective psyche with the latent numinosity attached to change.

The day upon which enquiry is made as to "what does psyche want?" is the day that the cure, if cure be intended, begins. Psyche has by way of the "symptom" endeavoured to indicate that the psychic libido is misdirected, deviated or obstructed. Something has gone awry, perhaps it is simply an error of judgment, a parental complex, the awakening of the anima, the presence of a destructive animus, or the advent of the Self into a life. A primitive mind would believe it was a visitation of the god. In any event, an old way has ended, and a new path is presenting itself. A death of the old, is to be superceded by a rebirth, or a renewal of the personality which has become imperative.

The crucial question to be asked regarding the advent of the disease, concerns time. It is essential to know exactly when it began, and it is of great interest to know what the subject did and thought at the time. This is called field thinking, and is opposite to lineal thinking. In the introduction to the Chinese book of Oracles the I Ching, Richard Wilhelm speaks of "a complex of events which occur at a certain moment". Von Franz[1] describes "synchronistic thinking as field thinking, the centre of which is time". In enlarging upon this theme, she says of synchronistic thinking,[2] "it is the classic way of thinking in China, thinking in fields. In Chinese philosophy such thinking has been developed and differentiated much more than in any other civilization: there the question is not, why has this come about, or what factor caused this effect, but what likes to happen together in a meaningful way in the same moment. The Chinese always ask 'What tends to happen together in time?' " So the centre of their field concept would be a time moment, on which are clustered the events.

Interestingly enough the subject is usually well aware of certain psychic events as soon as his attention is directed to the time factor.

The illness of the skin may thus be regarded as a message from the soul, the unconscious psyche of the subject. It is a warning that the conscious mind is unrelated to instinctive psyche, and has got out of touch with this inner world. If the message is heeded psychologically, a transformation usually occurs, and with the concomitant expansion of consciousness there is increased mental vitality and physical well being.

The hidden gift from the archetype of the Self, the archetype of order, is a healing of the dissociation, which is usually and rightly seen as an act of divine grace.

REFERENCES

1 Von Franz, M-L, On Divination and Synchronicity, p. 8, Inner City Books.
2 Ibid.

BIBLIOGRAPHY

Aschaffenberg, Gustav: Psychol., Arb (1896) p. 209-299 ll (1899) 1-82 IV (1904) 253-374.

Blum, Richard and Eva: The Dangerous Hour. Love and Culture Crisis in Ancient Greece. London: Chatto, 1970.

The Book of the Dead: Scribe and Treasures of the Temples of Egypt, About B.C. 1450. 2 Vols. Transl. and ed. By E. A. Wallis Budge. London. Philipp Lee Warner/New York: C. P. Putman's Sons, 1913.

Brown, Barbara B.: New Mind New Body. New York: Harper & Row, 1984.

Budge, E. A. Wallis: The Gods of the Egyptians. 2 Vols. New York: Dover Publications Inc., 1969.

Bunjes, W. E.: Medical and Pharmaceutical Dictionary. Stuttgart: Thieme, 1974.

Carus, Carl Gustav: Psyche. History of the Development of the Soul (1846) Jena, 1926.

Cumont, Franz: Die Mysterien des Mithra. Ein Beitrage zur Religionsgeschichte der römischen Kaiserzeit. Darmstadt: Wissenschaftliche Buchgesellschaft, 1975.

Eliade, Mircea: Shamanism. Archaic and Techniques of Ecstacy. 1951. Encyclopaedia of Religion and Ethics. Edinburgh: T. & T. Clarke 1914. Feldman, M., and Hugo A. J. Rondon, Psychosomatic Considerations in Alopecia Areata In: Med. Cut., Ibero. Lat. Amer. 7 (1973) p. 345–348.

Franz, Marie-Louise von: Animus, Inner Man in a Woman. In: Jung, C. G. Man and his Symbols Olten and and Freiburg im Breisgau: Walter, 1968.
Aurora Consurgens. In: C. G. Jung Collected Works Vol. 14, Pub. Bollingen Foundation 1963, U.S.A.
The Psychological Meaning of Redemption Motifs in Fairy Tales. 1980. Pub. Inner City Books.
The Problem of the Puer Aeturnus. 1970. Pub. Siga Sternback Scott. Sigo Press,

Patterns of Creativity Mirrored in Creation Myths, 1972.

On Divination and Synchronicity: The Psychology of Meaningful Chance. 1980. Pub. Inner City Books.

Frazer, J. G.: Folklore in the Old Testament. 3 Vols. London. Macmillan & Co., 1923.

The Golden Bough. A Study in Magic and Religion, 1927.

Friend, H.: Flowers and Flower Lore. 2 Vols. London: Swan and Sonnenshein & Co., 1883.

Galton, Francis: Psychometric Experiments. In: Brain 2 (1897), p. 149–162.

Hannah, Barbara: C. G. Jung, His Life and Work. Pub. By Putnam. New York and Longman Canada Ltd., 1976.

Herodot: Historien, Stuttgart: Kröner 1971.

Jung, C. C.: (Alchemy I and II) Modern Psychology. Lectures given at the ETH Zürich by Prof. C. G. Jung, 6 Vols. Darin. Bd. V: The Process of Individuation: Alchemy I (8 Nov 1940–28 Febr. 1941); Bd. VI: The Process of Individuation: Alchemy II (2. May–11 July 1941) Zürich. Karl Schippert & Co. 1960.

Letters 2 Vols., Walter, 1972.

Collected Works 20 Vols., Walter 1971.

C. G. Jung Speaking. Interviews and Encounters. Ed. By Wm. McQuire and R. E. C. Hull. U. S. A. Princeton, N. J. Princeton University Press, 1977.

The Visions Seminars. From the Complete Notes of Mary Foote, Postscript by Henry A. Murray, 2 Vols. Zürich; Spring Publications, 1976.

C. G. Jung Speaking. Hrsg. Von William McQuire, Princeton University Press., 1977.

Kraepelin, Emil: Experimental Studies of Association. Freiburg im Bresgau, 1883.

Layard, John: Making of Man in Malekula. In: Eranos Yearbook, 1948.

Lurker, Manfred: The Gods and Symbols of Ancient Egypt. Thames & Hudson, London, 1974.

Maguire, Anne; Psychic Possession Among Industrial Workers. In: The Lancet. (1978) p. 376–378.

The Crowned Serpent. In: Contribution to Festschrift for the 75th Birthday of Marie-Louise von Franz. Victor Orenga Editores S. L. 1991, p. 99–109.

Murray, M. A.: The God of the Witches. Oxford: Oxford University Press, 1952.

Macalpine, I.: Is Alopecia Areata Psychosomatic? In: British Journal of Dermatology 70 (1958).

The Mythology of All Races. 13 Vols., ed. By Canon John Arnott MacCulloch, New York: Macmillan Co. 1959.

Ogam: Traditional Celtique 12. Rennes 1948 p. 452-458.

Onians, Richard B.: Origins of European Thought. Cambridge: Cambridge University Press 1951-1988.

Ovidus Naso, Publius: Metamorphosen (lat. -dt). In deutsche Hexameter übertragen und mit dem Text hrsg. Von Erich Rösch. München und Zürich: Artemis 1983.

Rook, A., Wilkinson, D. S., and F. J. Ebling: Textbook of Dermatology, Oxford: Blackwell, 3. Aufl. 1979.

Servièr, J.: L'Homme et L'Invisible. Paris, 1964.

Shorter Oxford English Dictionary. Oxford: Oxford University Press, 1933.

Spearman, R. I. C.: The Keratinization of Epidermal Scales, Feathers, and Hairs. In: Biological Reviews 41, February 1966.

Tarchanoff, J.: Über die galvanischen Erscheinungen an der Haut des Menschen bei Reizungen der Sinnesorgane und bei verschiedenen Formen der psychischen Tätigkeit. In: (Pflüger's) Archiv für die gesamte Psychologie XLVI (Bonn u. Leipzig 1890), p. 46–55.

Veraguth, Otto: Le Réflexe psycho-galvanique. In: Archives de psychologie de la Suisse romande VI (Genf 1907), S. 162–163.

Windisch, Wilhelm: Irische Texte. 5 Vols. Leipzig 1880-1905 passim.

Wundt, Wilhelm: Sind die Mittelglieder einer mittelbaren Assoziation bewußt oder unbewußt? In: Philosophische Studien X (Leipzig 1892), S. 326-328.

GLOSSARY OF SPECIALIZED
TECHNICAL TERMS

Acantholytic: From the Greek Acantha – thorn. Skin disease with atrophy of the prickle cell layer in the epidermis.

Aetiology: The science or study of the causes of disease.

Alopecia: Loss of hair.

Anamnesis: Recall of things past.

Atopy: A dermatosis associated with familial hypersensitivities; hay fever, asthma.

Basal layer: Inner cell layer of the epidermis.

Collagenous: Appertaining to Connective tissue disease.

Corium: Deep layer of the skin. Cutis Vera or derma.

Dermatitis: Inflammation of the skin.

Dermatology: The science or the study of disorders of the skin.

Dermatosis: Any disease of the skin.

Dermis: Inner layer of the skin.

Diathesis: Constitution hereditary influence. A combination of attributes in an individual causing a susceptibility to disease.

Efflorescence: An eruption upon the skin, usually of a florid nature.

Eczema: An acute or chronic non-contagious itching, inflammatory disease of the skin.

Epidermis: Outer layer of the skin.

Exanthema: An eruption upon the skin.

Excoriation: Abrasion of a portion of the skin.

Exudate: The material exuded through vessel walls into adjacent tissues in inflammation.

Furor: Dermaticus Furiously angry and reddened skin with intense irritation.

Generalised: The extension of a primary lesion to other other parts of the body.

Histopathology: The study of minute changes in diseased tissue.

Integument: The skin.

206

Intraepidermal: Within the epidermal layer.

Irritation: Itching of the skin.

Keratin: Protein composition of horny tissues.

Keratosis: Any disease of the skin characterised by overgrowth of horny skin.

Lividity: Purple colour of the skin. Livid.

Localised: A disease process confined to one area.

Necrosis: Degeneration of tissue due to disease.

Oedema: Swelling of tissues due to accumulation of fluid in the tissue spaces.

Parakeratosis: Retention of nuclei in the horny layer ofskin.

Participation mystique: Is the term often used to denote that state which is none other than an unconscious identity or mutual unconscious relationship.

Perioral eczema: Eczema surrounding the mouth.

Proliferation: Increased expansion of eruption.

Subepidermal: Below the outer layer.

Tonus: The tone of the skin.

INDEX

Panther 32
Parents 62, 66ff, 69, 126, 132ff
Parental, complex 201
Pemphigus Vulgaris 11, 148–151
Penis 115, 116
Persona 103, 111, 137, 159
Personal, unconscious 15ff, 21
Personality, development of, 152
Petrification 163, 166, 167
Phallus 115
Phlogiston 178
Plague 113
Plateau, Phase, Illness 135
Polar Bear 51
Possession 65, 119
Pregnancy 145, 148, 151
Premature birth 148
Primitive Mind 200
Pride 20
Projection, unconscious 81, 155, 178
Prometheus 181
Protection 102, 156
Protein 156
Provisional Life 70
Pruritus 11
Psoriasis 11, 27, 92–106
Psyche 14ff, 19, 22, 148, 164, 201
  collective 95
  objective 22
Psychic Disorder 200
Psychopompos 166
Psychosis 122, 151, 194
  skin 156
Psychosomatic 17f, 125, 164
Psychic energy, libido 175, 201
Psychological Function 137ff
Puer Aeternus 69ff
Pulse rate, elevation 70
Python 106

Quaternio 195
Quaternity 148
Quetzal 38

Quetzalcoatl 185

Ra 31, 33
Ram 28, 31ff, 34ff
Rattlesnake 185
Rebirth renewal 201
Regeneration 176
Reindeer 148
Renewal 94, 181
Reptile 26, 46, 79, 8l, 93ff, 98, 106
Research 11ff
Respiratory problem 142
Revivification 182
Rheumatism 164
Rhinoceros 60
Ritual sacrifice 39
Rubbing 176–181
Rubedo 153, 159

Samothrace 40
Sanity, good health 196
Sarakka 148
Scalding 151
Scalping 42, 163
Scleroderma 11, 167-171
Sclerosis 167–169
Seed 164
Self (as Totality of Personality) 148, 201
  infliction 190
  mutilation 190
Shadow 68, 78, 119, 120, 137, 158ff, 188, 189
Shaman 148, 177
Shark 50
She-Devil 39, 139
Sheep 39
Schizophrenia 150
Serpent 27, 36, 38, 42, 50, 66, 68, 79–84, 91, 94, 95ff, 98, 102, 104, 128ff, 133, 164, 184, 196, 201
Serpent archetype 79ff, 175,

Unconscious, the 15ff, 17ff, 20, 21, 22, 23, 98, 180, 188, 189, 196, 200
Unity 60, 154
Urethral Orifice 115
Urticaria 11ff, 76–91, 122ff, 134, 187
  giant 88

Vesicular Diseases 134–154
Vesicular Eruption 11, 146, 149
Virgin Mary 85
Virus Infection 113
Volcano 55, 58, 70, 74, 140

Water, Hot 140

Wedding Ring 103
Weep, cry 113, 114
Willingness to serve 77
Wisdom 179
Wind 73
Witch 63, 103, 129, 131, 139
Wolf hound 166
Word Association Experiment 17–19, 161
Wotan 69

Xipe Totec 37 - 38

Youth 94

Zeus 34